GETTING STARTED

7 Containers = 1 Easy Solution 4
Calculate Your Calorie Target 6
Find the Portion Plan That's Right for You 10
Tally Sheets 14

USING THE CONTAINERS

Container Food Groups 18
Substitutions 28
Freebies 32
FAQ 38

RECIPES

Seasoning Mixes 42
Green Container 44
Red Container 46
Yellow Container 52
Dressings 58
Sweet Treats 64
Shakeology 68
Sample Portion Plan 72

INTRODUCTION

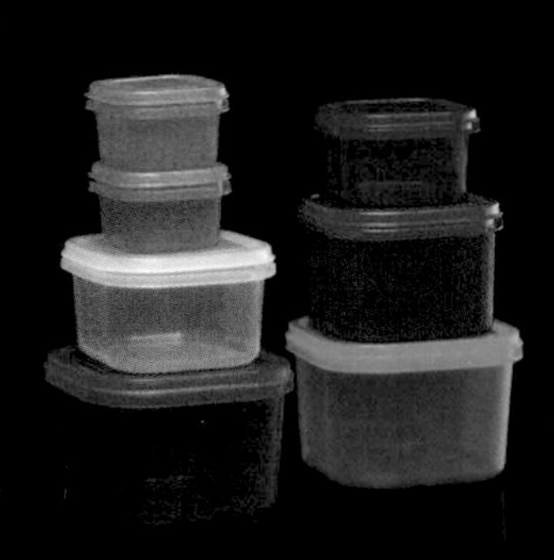

We all know that nutrition plays an incredibly important role in helping you achieve your weight-loss goals—that means eating healthy and maintaining proper portion sizes. With Portion Fix® you have a straightforward system to get portions right for weight loss and weight management.

Seven easy to use color-coded containers and a nutrient-rich food plan constructed around the proven balance of roughly 40% carbohydrates, 30% protein, and 30% fat, a balance that's great for either weight loss or maintaining your current healthy lifestyle.

In this guide, you'll find three sections that tell you everything you need to know to begin using your Portion Fix containers, along with healthy and delicious recipes! Simple, easy, and totally foolproof.

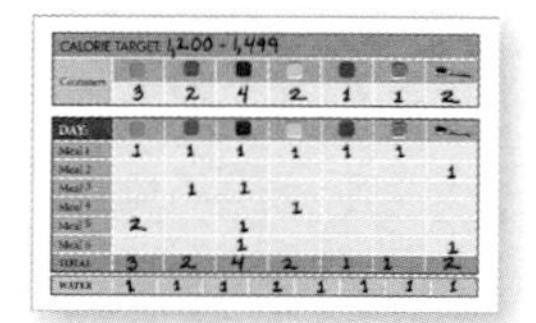

GETTING STARTED

You'll learn how the Portion Fix containers work and how to calculate your Calorie Target to find the right Portion Plan for you. There is a little "calorie math" in the beginning to avoid a lot of math every day. You'll also find Tally Sheets here that will help you keep track of your portions daily!

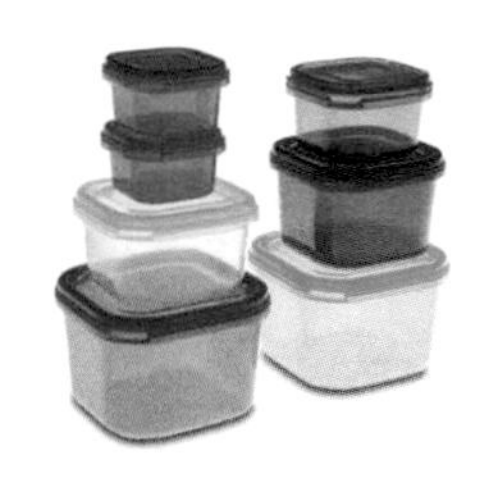

USING THE CONTAINERS

Everything you need to know about using the seven color-coded containers, including Food Lists, food substitutions, free foods, and Frequently Asked Questions.

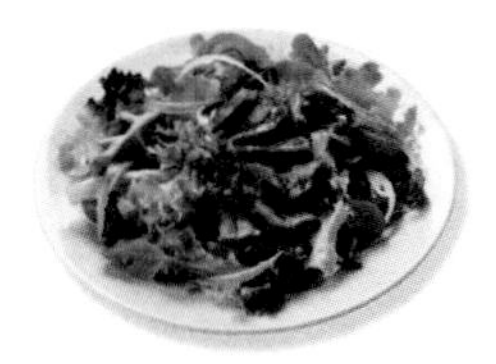

RECIPES

Delicious, healthy recipes designed to work perfectly with the Portion Fix containers along with a simple-to-follow sample 3-day Portion Plan.

7 CONTAINERS =

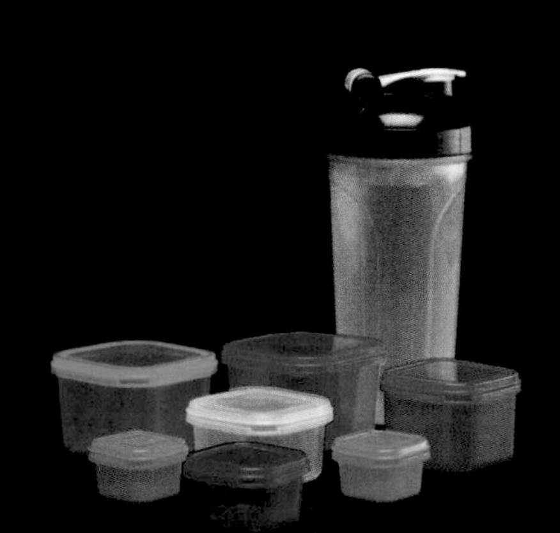

The key to success with the Portion Fix are the **7** containers and Shakeology® shaker cup that came with this guide. You'll use these containers to portion and transport all of your meals.

1 EASY SOLUTION

These little squares in the Portion Plan correspond with the food container of the same color.

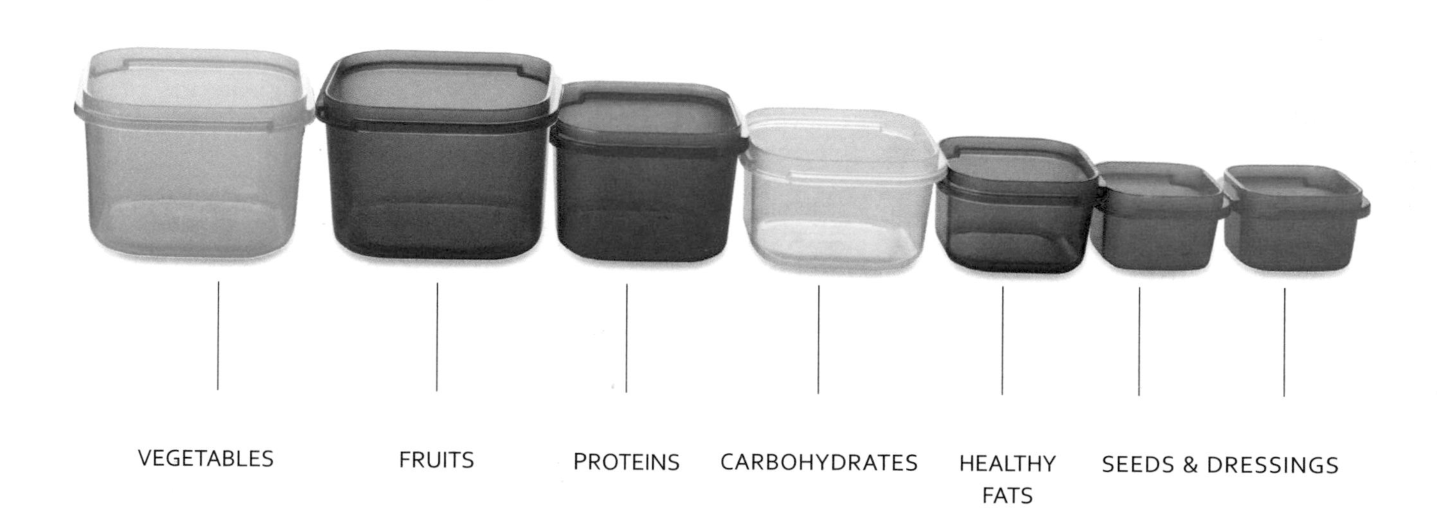

GETTING STARTED

This is where it begins, and you're about to get some incredible results. Let's get started!

1. Find your CALORIE TARGET for weight loss.
2. Then use your Calorie Target to find the corresponding PORTION PLAN.

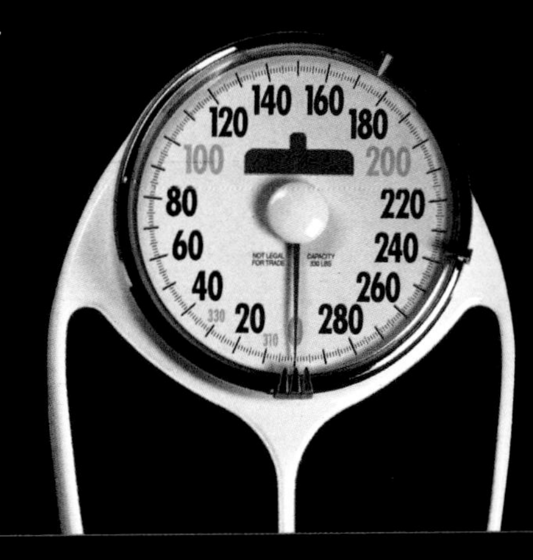

1 CALCULATE YOUR CALORIE TARGET

You can find your Calorie Target with some very simple math:

A

First, find your **Caloric Baseline** (approximately how many calories you burn in a day). To do that you'll first need to determine whether your lifestyle is considered "sedentary," "moderately active," or "highly active." See below:

	SEDENTARY LIFESTYLE	MODERATELY ACTIVE LIFESTYLE	HIGHLY ACTIVE LIFESTYLE
If you:	• have a desk job • watch a lot of TV • never take the stairs	• have a desk job but try to stay active and on your feet • work out occasionally • take the stairs instead of the elevator	• have a physical job • move as much as you can
Then do this to find your Caloric Baseline:	______ x 11 = ______ Current Weight (lbs.) / Caloric Baseline	______ x 12 = ______ Current Weight (lbs.) / Caloric Baseline	______ x 13 = ______ Current Weight (lbs.) / Caloric Baseline

B | Then use your Caloric Baseline to find your **Maintenance Calories**. To do that you'll need to determine whether your exercise program/regimen is "moderately challenging" or "extremely challenging." See below:

	MODERATELY CHALLENGING	EXTREMELY CHALLENGING
If you do:	• Yoga • Easy jogging • PiYO • P90 • 21 day FIX • 10 Minute Trainer • Leandro Carvalho's Brazil Butt Lift • Focus T25 • tai CHENG • Slim in 6 • turbo jam • Hip Hop Abs • Rockin' Body	• Long-distance running or intense intervals • Mixed martial arts • P90X • P90X2 • P90X3 • Body Beast • INSANITY • INSANITY THE ASYLUM • INSANITY MAX:30 • 21 day FIX EXTREME • TURBO FIRE • CHALEAN EXTREME
Then do this to find your Maintenance Calories:	________ (Caloric Baseline) + 400 = ________ (Maintenance Calories)	________ (Caloric Baseline) + 700 = ________ (Maintenance Calories)

C | Finally, let's calculate your **Calorie Target** for weight loss.

____________________ - 750 = ____________________

Your Maintenance Calories — Your Calorie Target

IMPORTANT TIPS:

- *If you want to maintain weight, stick with your **Maintenance Calories***
- *If you want to gain weight, add 350 calories to your **Maintenance Calories***
- *If your **Calorie Target** is less than 1,200, round up to 1,200*
- *If your **Calorie Target** is more than 2,800, round down to 2,800*

NOTE: There are many variables to this, so you can refine these numbers to your specific situation and goals, just make sure you do not *under-eat*.

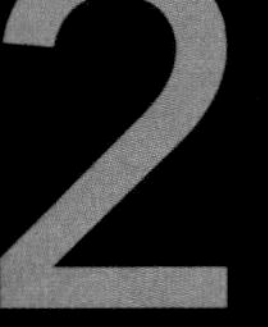

FIND THE PORTION PLAN THAT'S RIGHT FOR YOU

Now just use your Calorie Target to find the customized **Portion Plan** for your specific weight-loss needs.

Each plan is color-coded to match the 7 containers, with the number of portions per container listed next to the colored square. For example, if you have a "3" next to the Yellow square, that means you'll be filling the Yellow Container three times a day.

The plans also include daily teaspoon-sized portions of oils and/or nut butters—just look for the symbol in your Portion Plan. The Portion Fix doesn't include an actual teaspoon, so just use any standard teaspoon.

Healthy foods, like fruits, veggies, and lean proteins, tend to have a lot more volume than fried or sugary foods, so at first the amount of food on your plate may seem overwhelming. You don't need to eat it all if you get full. You just need to make sure you're feeding your body ENOUGH to support your metabolism and get the appropriate macronutrients.

At any meal, you can just eat the amount that feels right. In time, your appetite will adapt to this more "natural" way of balanced eating throughout the day.

THE PORTION PLANS

IF YOUR CALORIE TARGET FALLS BETWEEN 1,200 – 1,499 CALORIES	
PORTION PLAN A	
VEGETABLES	3
FRUITS	2
PROTEINS	4
CARBOHYDRATES	2
HEALTHY FATS	1
SEEDS & DRESSINGS	1
OILS & NUT BUTTERS	2

IF YOUR CALORIE TARGET FALLS BETWEEN 1,500 – 1,799 CALORIES	
PORTION PLAN B	
VEGETABLES	4
FRUITS	3
PROTEINS	4
CARBOHYDRATES	3
HEALTHY FATS	1
SEEDS & DRESSINGS	1
OILS & NUT BUTTERS	4

IF YOUR CALORIE TARGET FALLS BETWEEN 1,800 – 2,099 CALORIES

PORTION PLAN C

VEGETABLES	5
FRUITS	3
PROTEINS	5
CARBOHYDRATES	4
HEALTHY FATS	1
SEEDS & DRESSINGS	1
OILS & NUT BUTTERS	5

IF YOUR CALORIE TARGET FALLS BETWEEN 2,100 – 2,299 CALORIES

PORTION PLAN D

VEGETABLES	6
FRUITS	4
PROTEINS	6
CARBOHYDRATES	4
HEALTHY FATS	1
SEEDS & DRESSINGS	1
OILS & NUT BUTTERS	6

IF YOUR CALORIE TARGET FALLS BETWEEN
2,300 – 2,499 CALORIES

PORTION PLAN E

VEGETABLES		7
FRUITS		5
PROTEINS		6
CARBOHYDRATES		5
HEALTHY FATS		1
SEEDS & DRESSINGS		1
OILS & NUT BUTTERS	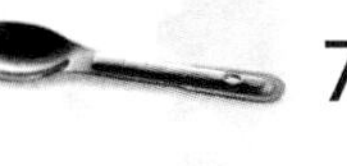	7

IF YOUR CALORIE TARGET FALLS BETWEEN
2,500 – 2,800 CALORIES

PORTION PLAN F

VEGETABLES		8
FRUITS		5
PROTEINS		7
CARBOHYDRATES		5
HEALTHY FATS		1
SEEDS & DRESSINGS		1
OILS & NUT BUTTERS		8

TALLY SHEETS

The following pages contain 4 days of Tally Sheets to keep track of your daily food intake.

Be sure to make additional copies of the tally sheets for food planning before you fill these in! You can also find a copy of the Tally Sheets at TeamBeachbody.com under GET FIT > FITNESS TOOLS > WORKOUT SHEETS.

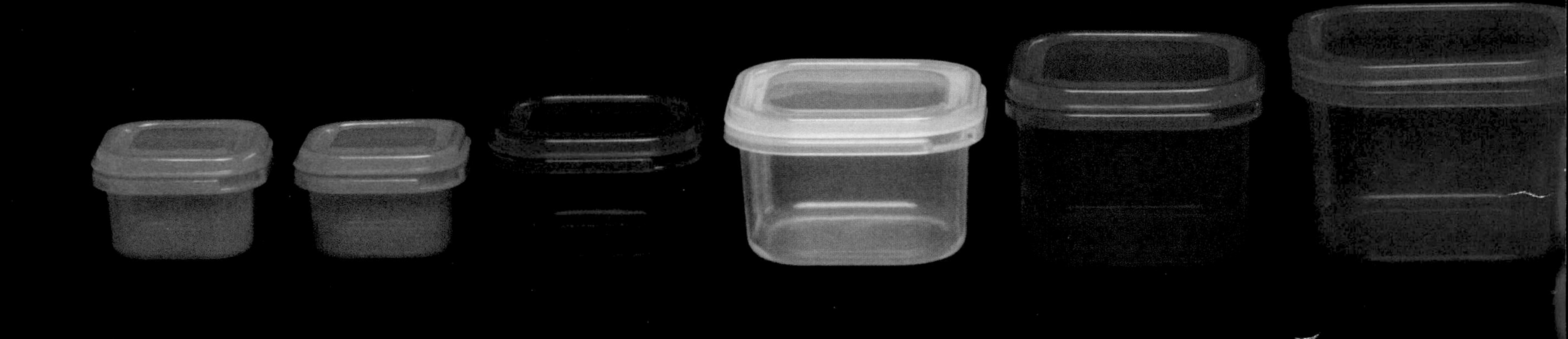

To use the Tally Sheets, just fill in the top row after "Containers" with your Portion Plan allotment. Then fill in the squares below it as you eat your daily meals.

And don't forget to hydrate! (That's why we've provided the eight water slots at the bottom of each day.)

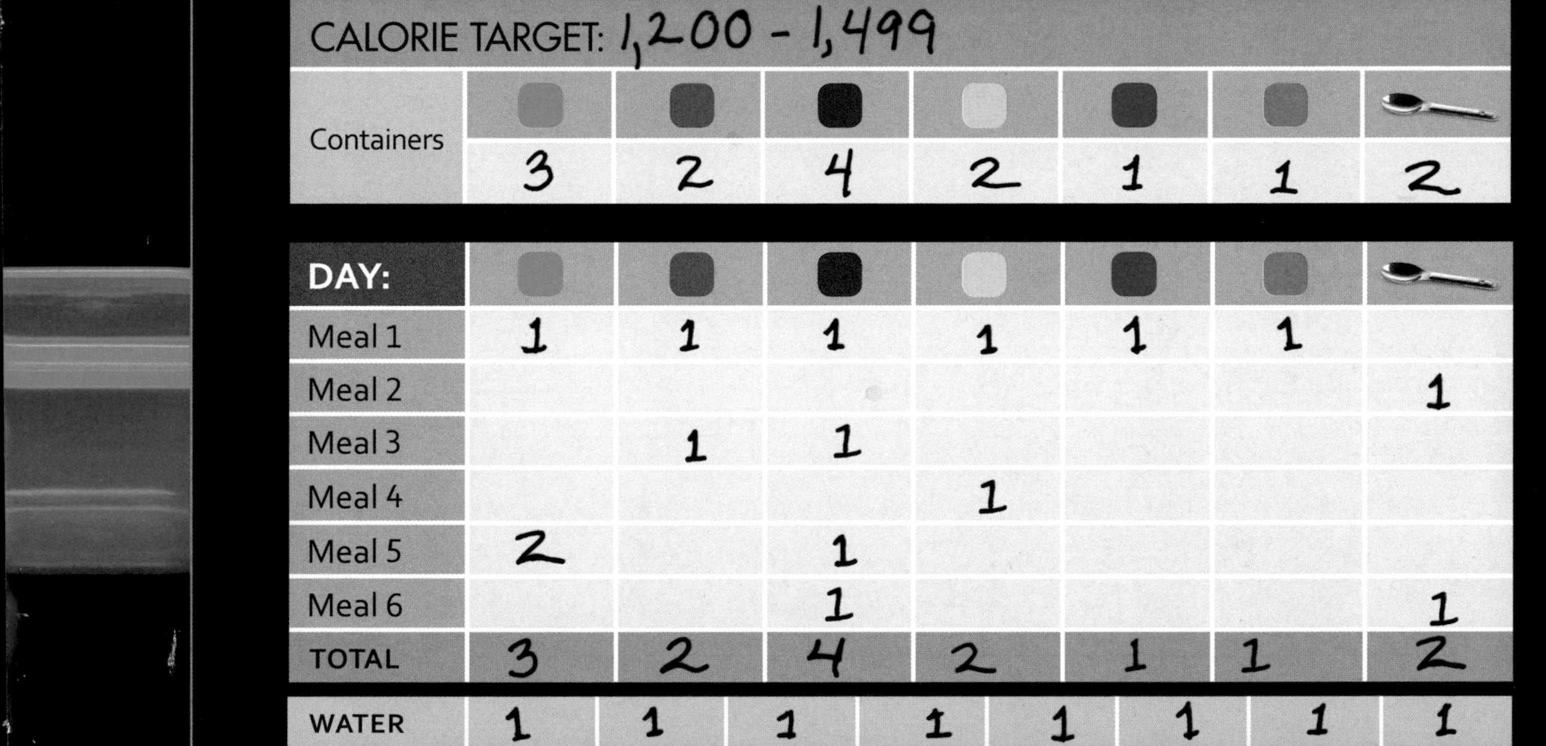

CALORIE TARGET: 1,200 - 1,499							
Containers	3	2	4	2	1	1	2

DAY:							
Meal 1	1	1	1	1	1	1	
Meal 2							1
Meal 3		1	1				
Meal 4				1			
Meal 5	2		1				
Meal 6			1				1
TOTAL	3	2	4	2	1	1	2

WATER	1	1	1	1	1	1	1	1

Remember to copy these tally sheets before filling them in or go to TeamBeachbody.com under GET FIT > FITNESS TOOLS > WORKOUT SHEETS.

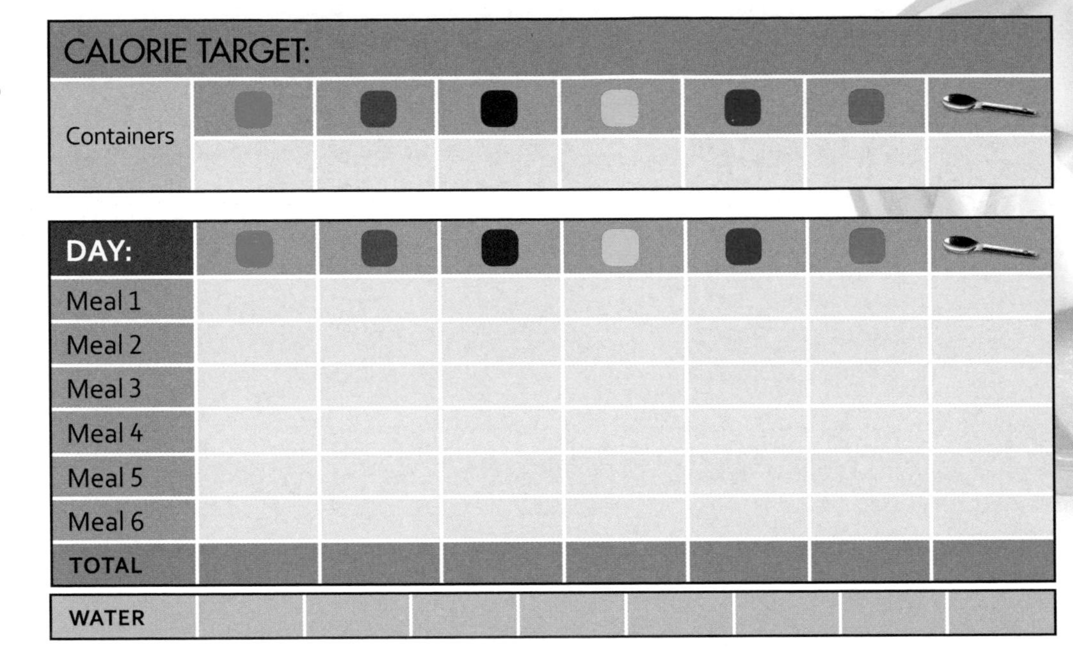

CALORIE TARGET:							
Containers							

DAY:							
Meal 1							
Meal 2							
Meal 3							
Meal 4							
Meal 5							
Meal 6							
TOTAL							

WATER								

DAY:							
Meal 1							
Meal 2							
Meal 3							
Meal 4							
Meal 5							
Meal 6							
TOTAL							

WATER								

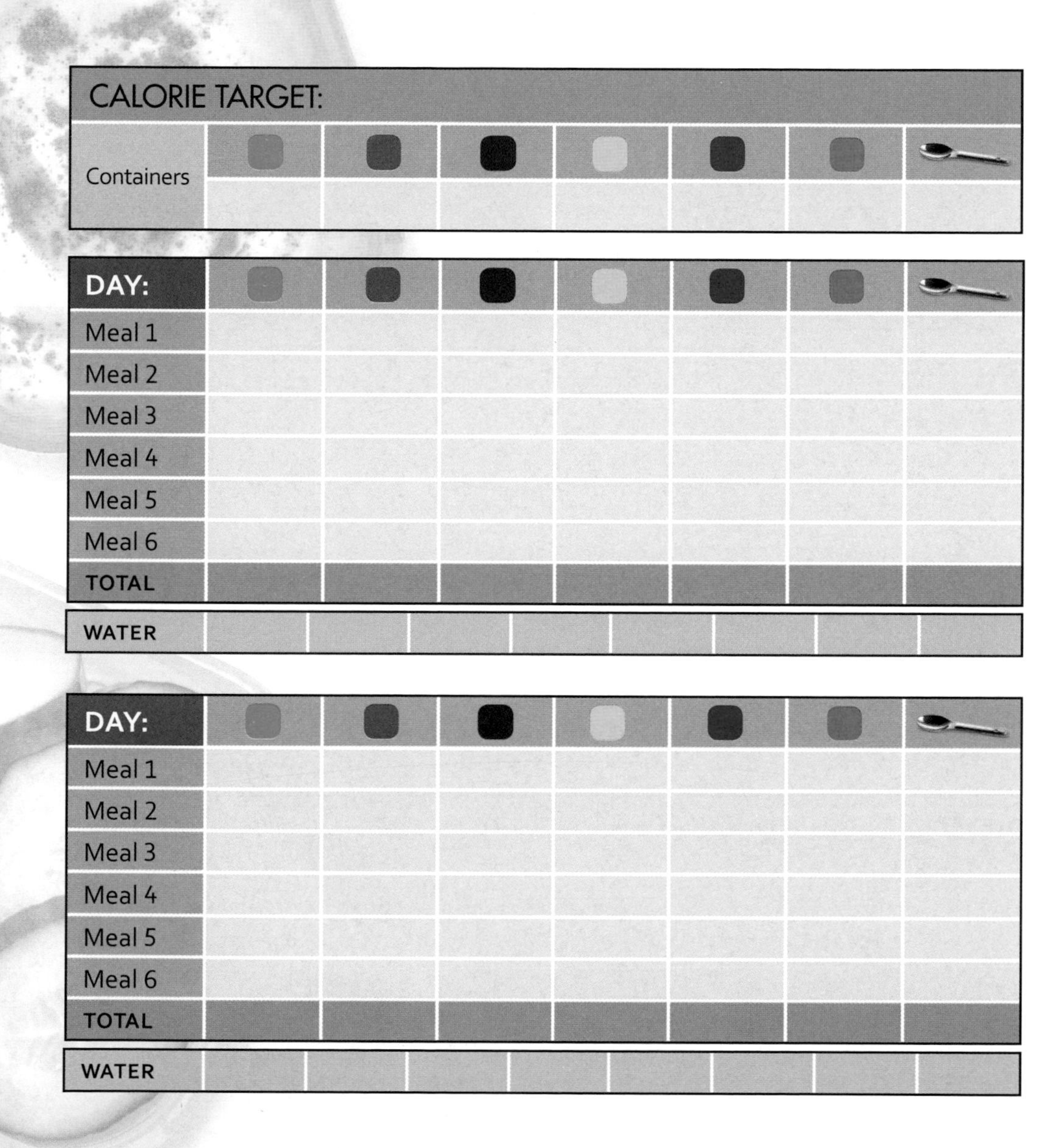

CALORIE TARGET:							
Containers							

DAY:							
Meal 1							
Meal 2							
Meal 3							
Meal 4							
Meal 5							
Meal 6							
TOTAL							

WATER								

DAY:							
Meal 1							
Meal 2							
Meal 3							
Meal 4							
Meal 5							
Meal 6							
TOTAL							

WATER								

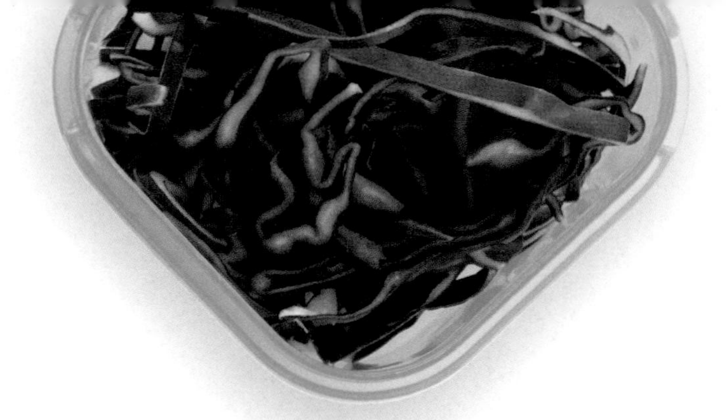

CONTAINER FOOD GROUPS

Now that you have found your individual Portion Plan, all you need to do is fill the containers with the allowed foods for each Portion Fix container and plan your meals. A few important things to note before you get started:

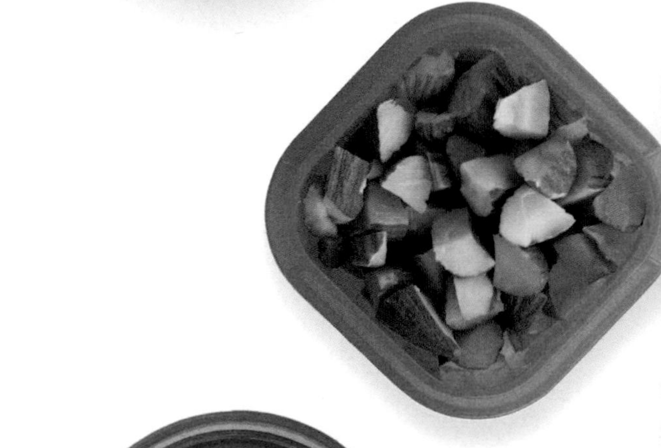

- The foods are arranged by each color-coded container, and according to nutritional value—the higher up on the list, the more nutritionally beneficial the food! But you shouldn't ignore the foods lower down the list, it's important that your body gets a large variety of nutrients.

- Most of the foods are listed with specific measurements/amounts—10 asparagus spears, for example. But if there's no amount, just fill the container to the point that you can still fit the lid on it.

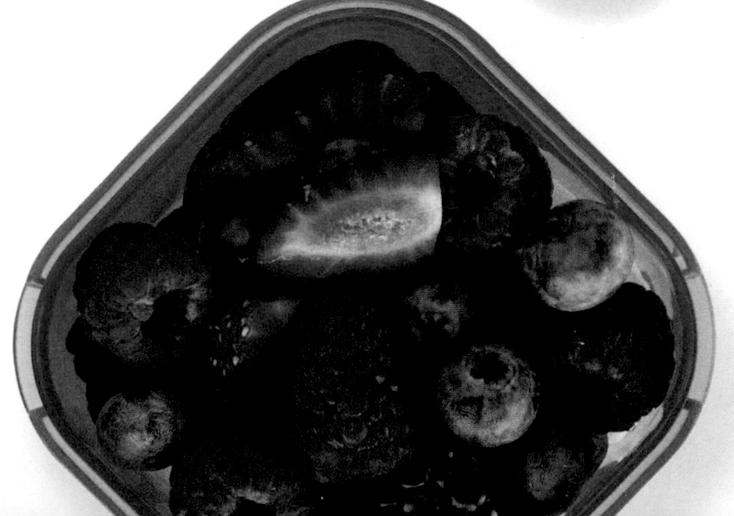

The container categories are based on food groups (vegetables, fruits, etc.) AND macronutrient groups (fats, proteins, and carbohydrates). We do this to make sure that you're getting the right balance of vitamins, minerals, phytonutrients, *and* macronutrients for a healthy diet. Since many foods can feature different combinations of these macronutrients, we've categorized these complex foods based on how their macronutrient level best fits into the Portion Fix Eating Plan.

STRATEGY FOR STAYING ON TRACK

It's a great idea to transfer the food to your own plates, bowls, or larger containers so you'll be better able to "eyeball" what healthy portions should look like. We've noticed that portions tend to expand over time with just the "eyeball" method, so keep the containers for a good refresher when you start to see your progress going in the other direction.

GREEN
CONTAINER (Vegetables)

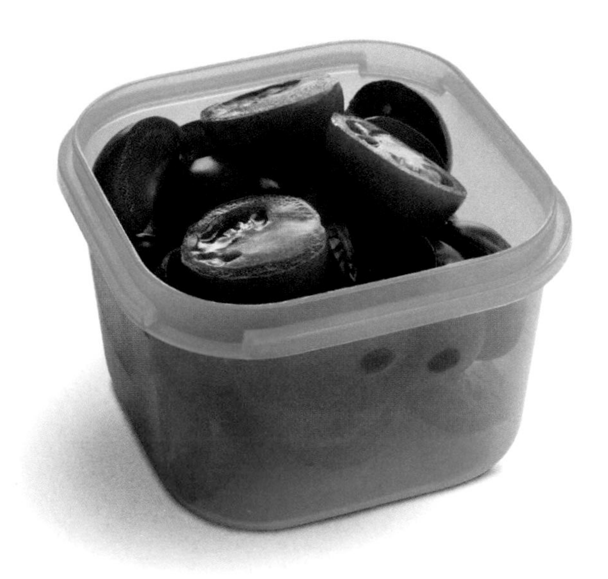

- Kale, cooked or raw
- Collard greens, cooked or raw
- Spinach, cooked or raw
- Brussels sprouts, chopped or 5 medium
- Broccoli, chopped
- Asparagus, 10 large spears
- Beets, 2 medium
- Tomatoes, chopped, cherry, or 2 medium
- Squash (summer), sliced
- Winter squash (all varieties), cubed
- String beans
- Peppers, sweet, sliced
- Carrots, sliced or 10 medium baby
- Cauliflower, chopped
- Artichokes, ½ large
- Eggplant, ½ medium
- Okra
- Jicama, sliced
- Snow peas
- Cabbage, chopped
- Cucumbers
- Celery
- Lettuce (NOT iceberg)
- Mushrooms
- Radishes
- Onions, chopped
- Sprouts

PURPLE
CONTAINER (Fruits)

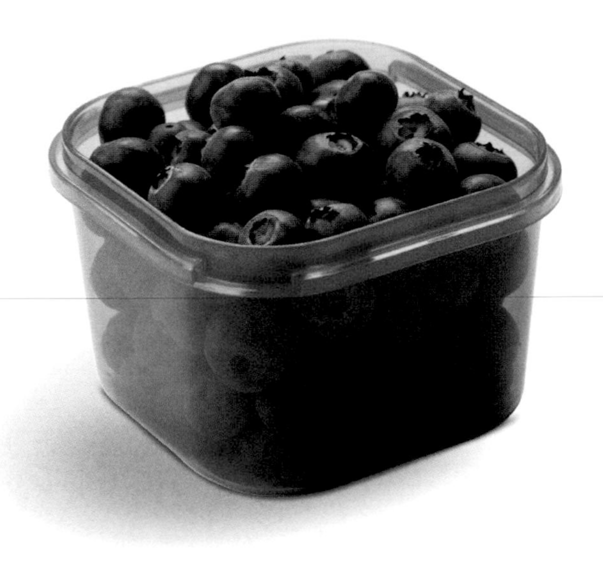

- Raspberries
- Blueberries
- Blackberries
- Strawberries
- Watermelon, diced
- Cantaloupe, diced
- Orange, divided into sections or 1 medium
- Tangerine, 2 small
- Apple, sliced or 1 small
- Apricots, 4 small
- Grapefruit, divided into sections or ½ large
- Cherries
- Grapes
- Kiwifruit, 2 medium
- Mango, sliced
- Peach, sliced or 1 large
- Nectarine, sliced or 1 large
- Pear, sliced or 1 large
- Pineapple, diced
- Banana, ½ large
- Papaya, diced
- Figs, 2 small
- Honeydew melon, diced
- Salsa, pico de gallo
- Tomato sauce, plain

RED
CONTAINER (Proteins)

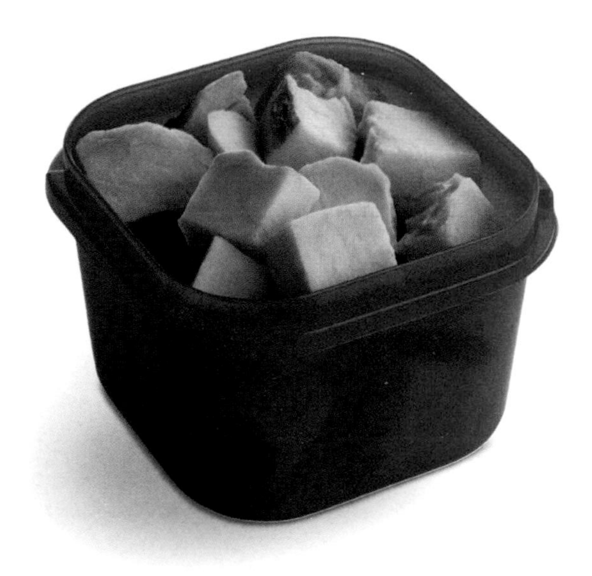

A NOTE ABOUT EGGS:
Generally we recommend eating whole eggs because the yolk is so nutrient-dense. Egg whites only can be eaten when you're trying to increase protein intake but not fat intake, but that type of situation is a rare exception.

- Sardines (fresh or canned in water), 7 medium
- Boneless, skinless chicken or turkey breast, cooked, diced
- Lean ground chicken or turkey (≥ 93% lean), cooked
- Fish, fresh water (catfish, tilapia, trout), cooked, flaked
- Fish, cold water, wild-caught (cod, salmon, halibut, tuna), cooked, flaked
- Game: buffalo (bison, ostrich, venison), cooked, diced
- Game: lean ground (≥ 95% lean), cooked, diced
- Eggs, 2 large
- Egg whites, 8 large
- Greek yogurt, plain, 1%
- Yogurt, plain, 2%
- Shellfish (shrimp, crab, lobster), cooked
- Clams, canned, drained
- Red meat, extra-lean, cooked, diced
- Lean ground red meat (≥ 95% lean), cooked
- Shakeology, 1 scoop
- Tempeh
- Tofu, firm
- Pork tenderloin, diced, cooked
- Tuna, canned light in water, drained
- Turkey slices, low-sodium, fat-free, 6 slices
- Ham slices, low-sodium, fat-free, 6 slices
- Ricotta cheese, light
- Cottage cheese, 2%
- Protein powder (whey, hemp, rice, pea), 1½ scoops (approx. 42 g depending on variety)
- Veggie burger, 1 medium patty
- Turkey bacon (reduced fat), 4 slices

SHAKEOLOGY

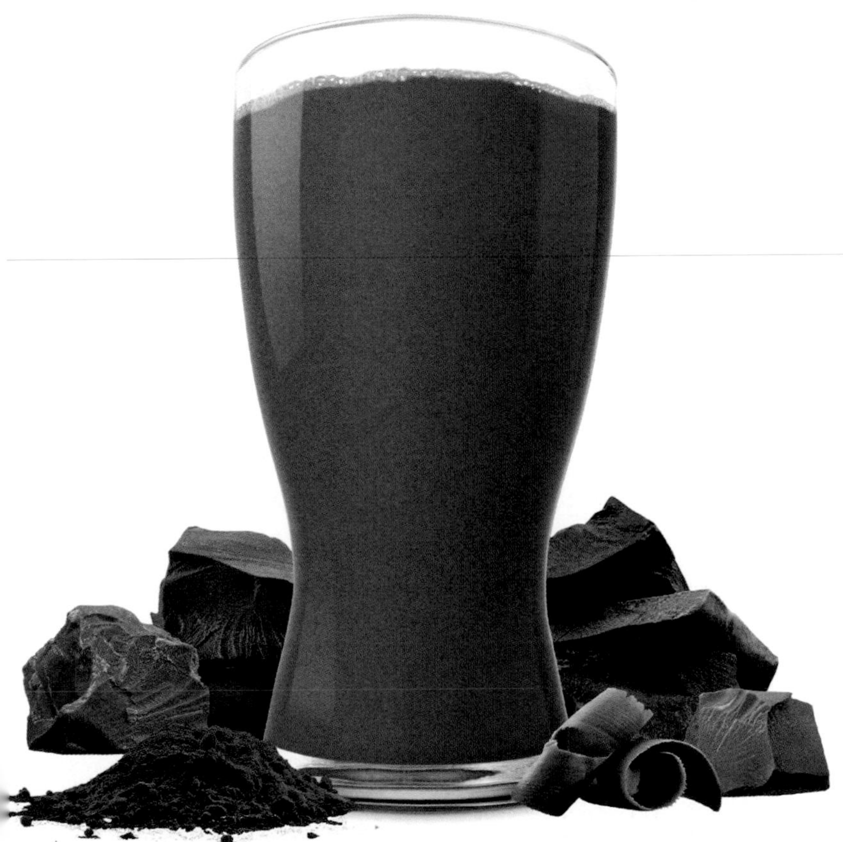

Beachbody® formulated this shake at the request of our CEO, who is a self-proclaimed "toddler" when it comes to eating his fruits and vegetables. Shakeology is Your Daily Dose of Dense Nutrition®, and we not only sell it, we drink it every single day. (Our company kitchen sounds like a blender testing lab.) We highly recommend this super-healthy, super-satisfying superfood shake as part of your Portion Fix if you want to lose weight, improve your energy, regularity, and help your body operate at its most healthy.* See page 68 for a great list of recipes showing you how to do just that.

Part of the reasoning behind weaving Shakeology into this program is the fact that when you reduce calories, you can miss out on important nutrients. Similarly, if you're doing an intense workout program, you're more likely to deplete your body of those nutrients—even if your diet is packed with healthy food. Drinking Shakeology daily is a powerful way to make sure you're not missing out on anything important. And quite honestly, it's delish.

*These statements have not been evaluated by the Food and Drug Administration. This product is not intended to diagnose, treat, cure, or prevent any disease.

YELLOW
CONTAINER (Carbohydrates)

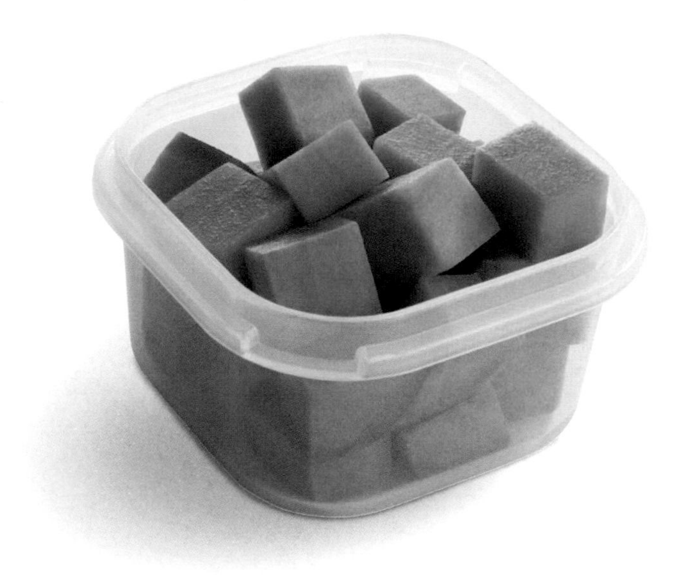

- Sweet potato
- Yams
- Quinoa, cooked
- Beans (kidney, black, garbanzo, white, lima, etc.), cooked, drained
- Lentils, cooked, drained
- Edamame, shelled
- Peas
- Refried beans, nonfat
- Brown rice, cooked
- Wild rice, cooked
- Potato, mashed or ½ medium
- Corn on the cob, 1 ear
- Amaranth, cooked
- Millet, cooked
- Buckwheat, cooked
- Barley, cooked
- Bulgur, cooked
- Oatmeal, steel-cut, cooked
- Oatmeal, rolled, cooked
- Pasta, whole-grain, cooked
- Couscous, whole wheat, cooked
- Crackers, whole-grain, 8 small crackers
- Cereal, whole-grain, low sugar
- Bread, whole-grain, 1 slice*
- Pita bread, whole wheat, 1 small (4-inch)*
- Waffles, whole-grain, 1 waffle*
- Pancakes, whole-grain, 1 small (4-inch)*
- English muffin, whole-grain, ½ muffin*
- Bagel, whole-grain, ½ small (3-inch)*
- Tortilla, whole wheat, 1 small (6-inch)*
- Tortilla, corn, 2 small (6-inch)*

* These food items don't fit in the containers, so just use the indicated amount.

BLUE
CONTAINER (Healthy Fats)

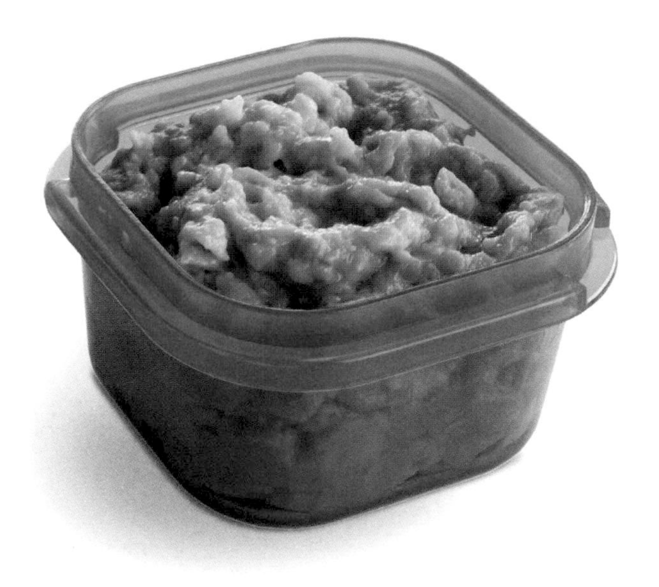

- Avocado, mashed or ¼ medium
- 12 almonds, whole, raw
- 8 cashews, whole, raw
- 14 peanuts, whole, raw
- 20 pistachios, whole, raw
- 10 pecan halves, raw
- 8 walnut halves, raw
- Hummus
- Coconut milk, canned
- Feta cheese, crumbled
- Goat cheese, crumbled
- Mozzarella (low-moisture), shredded
- Cheddar, shredded
- Provolone, shredded
- Monterey jack, shredded
- Parmesan, shredded

ORANGE
CONTAINER (Seeds & Dressings)

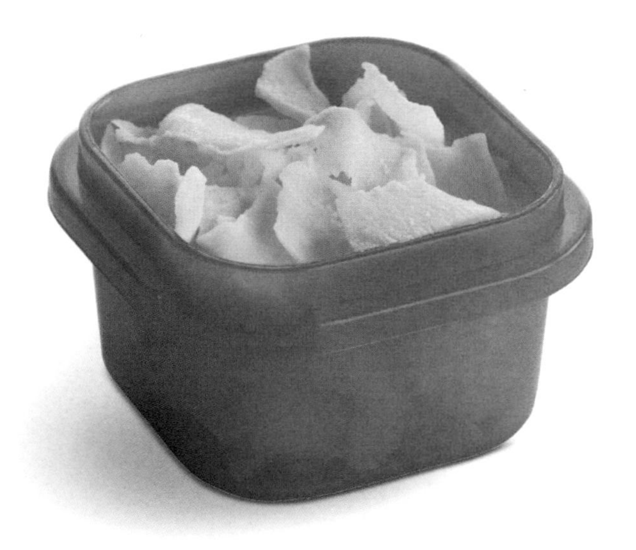

- Pumpkin seeds, raw
- Sunflower seeds, raw
- Sesame seeds, raw
- Flaxseed, ground
- Olives, 10 medium
- Peanuts
- Coconut, unsweetened, shredded
- PORTION FIX DRESSINGS (see page 58)

TEASPOON*
(Oils & Nut Butters)

- Extra-virgin olive oil
- Extra-virgin coconut oil
- Flaxseed oil
- Walnut oil
- Pumpkin seed oil
- Nut butters (peanut, almond, cashew, etc.)
- Seed butters (pumpkin, sunflower, sesame [tahini])

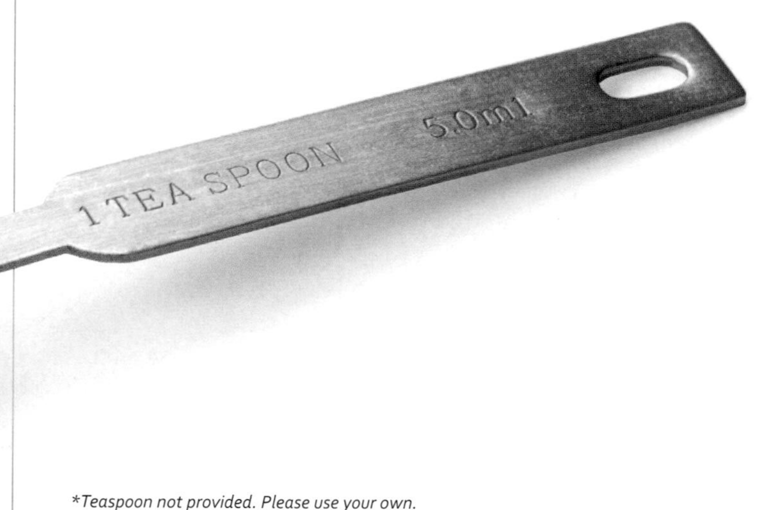

**Teaspoon not provided. Please use your own.*

SUBSTITUTIONS

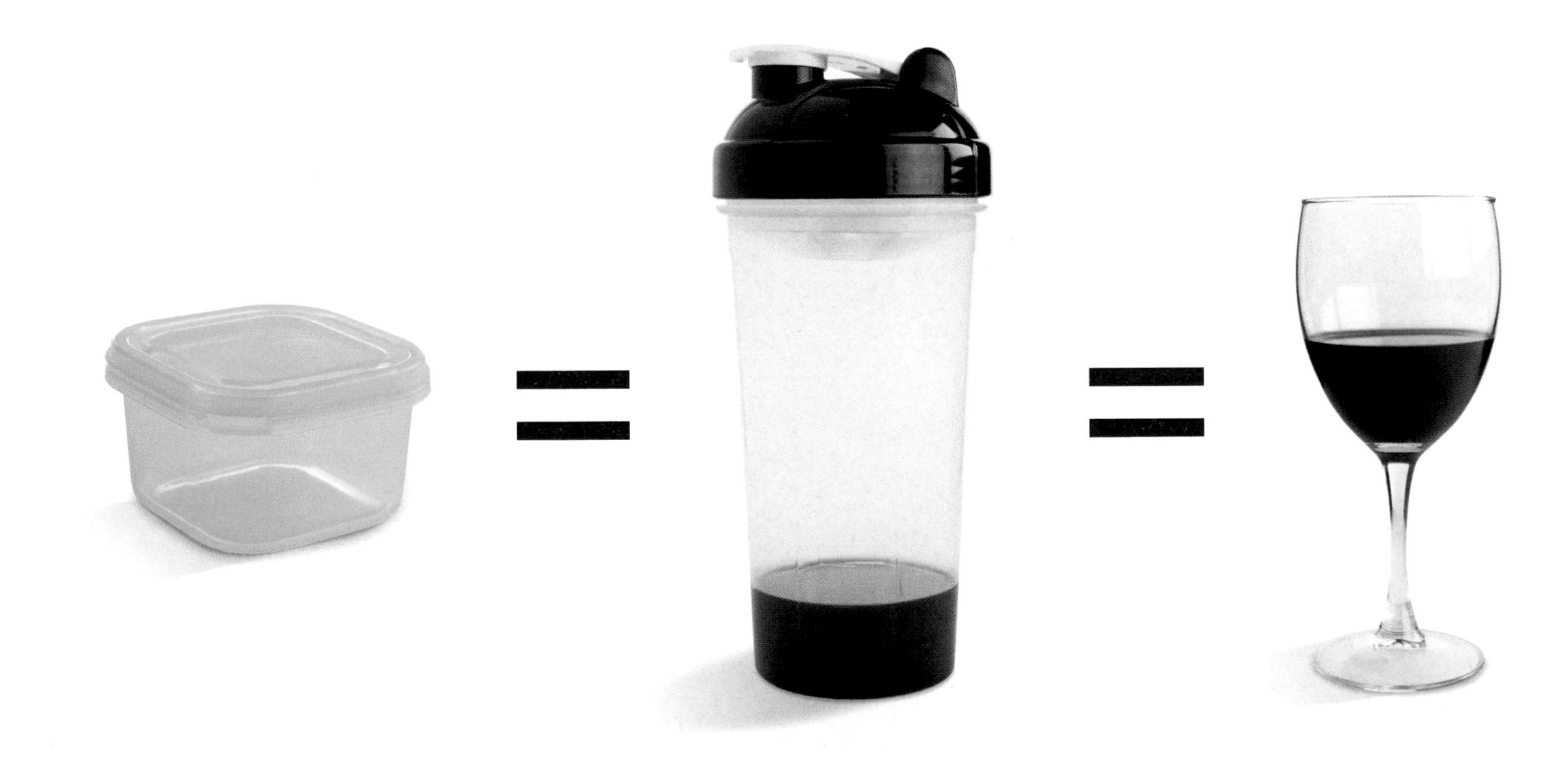

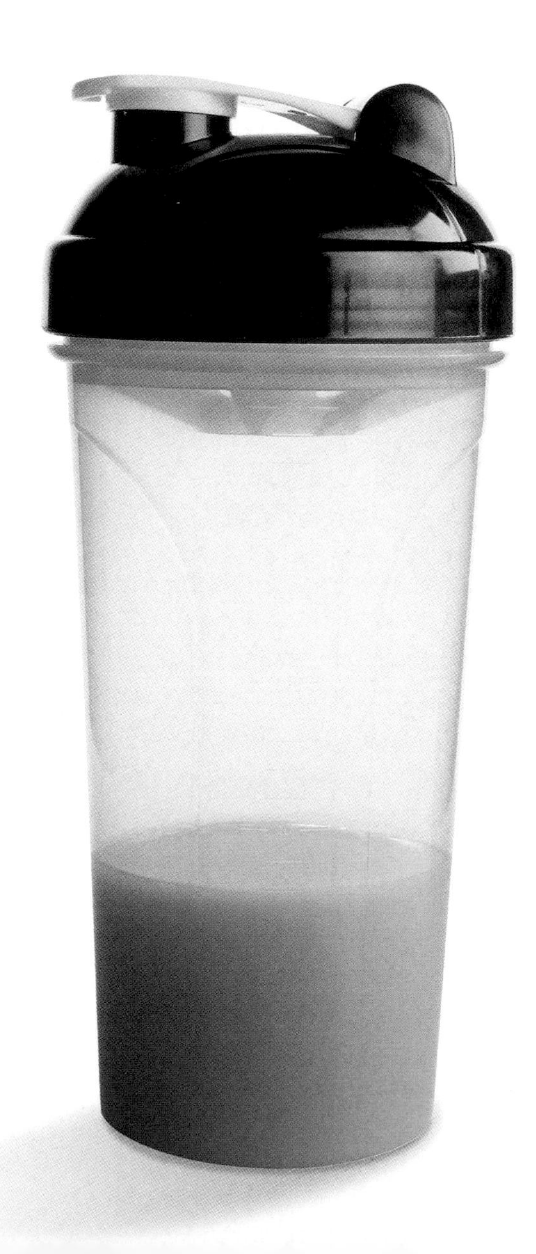

BEVERAGES

Three times a week, you can replace one of your Yellow Container portions with a beverage from the list below. To do this, fill the provided Shakeology shaker cup (not the Yellow Container) to the fluid ounce mark indicated below for that beverage and *check off a Yellow Container portion on your Tally Sheet.*

- Milk, cow's, nonfat or 1%, 8 fl oz
- Soy milk,
  unsweetened, 8 fl oz
  sweetened, 6 fl oz
- Almond milk,
  unsweetened, 16 fl oz
  sweetened, 8 fl oz
- Coconut water, 16 fl oz
- Coconut milk beverage (from a carton, not canned),
  unsweetened, 12 fl oz
  sweetened, 8 fl oz
- Fresh fruit juices, 8 fl oz
- Rice milk, original or vanilla, 6 fl oz
- Wine, 4 fl oz
- P90X Results and Recovery Formula®, 1 scoop (30 grams)*

**If your exercise level is extreme, you can replace two Yellow Containers so that you can have 2 scoops of Results and Recovery Formula—a full serving. Feel free to do this after any intense workout, not just three times a week.*

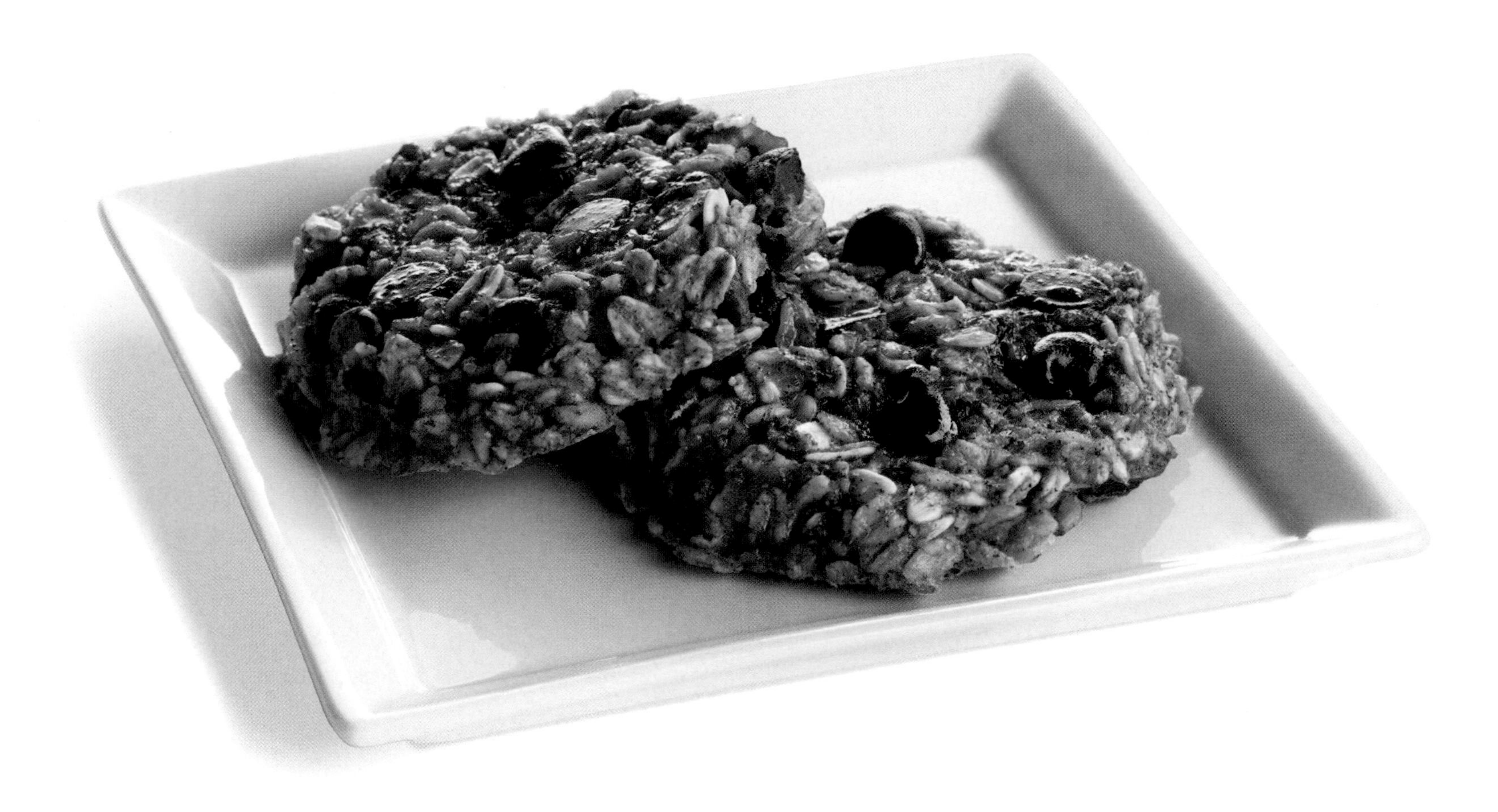

TREATS

You can also replace a Yellow Container with a treat three times a week. Just use the matching container (orange container, yellow container, or teaspoon) next to the treat of your choice to measure your treat. *However, you'll still check a Yellow Container off your Tally Sheet.*

For example, if you decide to indulge in a few well-earned chocolate-covered raisins, fill the Orange Container with your treat, but check a Yellow Container off your Tally Sheet.

- Dried fruit medley
- Chocolate chips or chunks, dark
- Potato chips, plain kettle
- Tortilla chips, plain corn
- Chocolate-covered raisins
- 6 Chocolate-covered almonds
- 2 Banana Oatmeal Cookies (see page 67)
- 1 Double Chocolate Cookie (see page 65)
- 2 Oatmeal Cookies with Chocolate Morsels and Toasted Pecans (see page 66)
- 1 High-Protein Chocolate Peanut Butter Snack Bar (see page 66)
- Popcorn Mix with Raisins, Almonds, and Dried Fruit (see page 64)

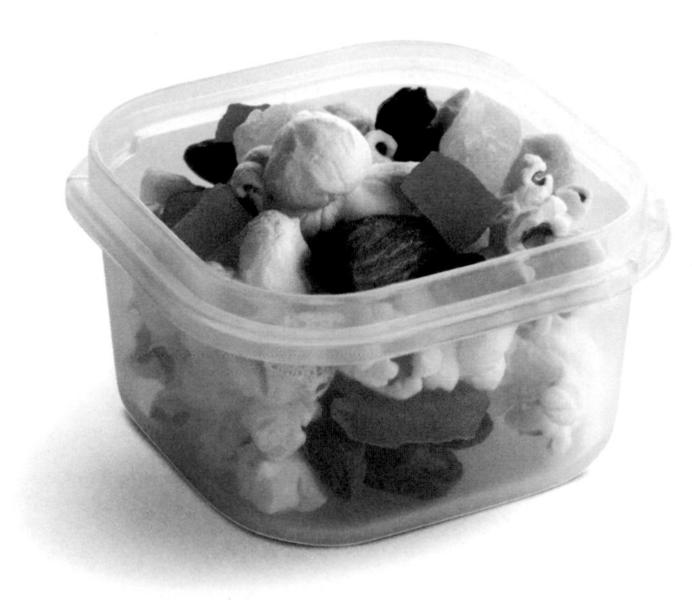

FREEBIES

WATER

Up to 60% of the human body is water. It plays a vital role in flushing toxins out of your system and delivering nutrients. And it helps you feel full—which is especially important when you're watching your portions.

We recommend you drink your body weight, divided by two, in ounces. So if you weigh 180 pounds, that would be 180 ÷ 2 = 90. That's 90 ounces of water, every day.

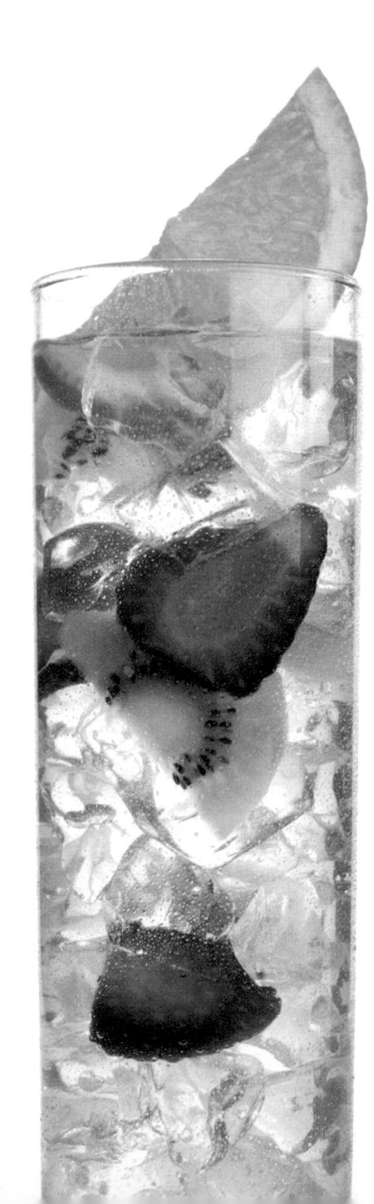

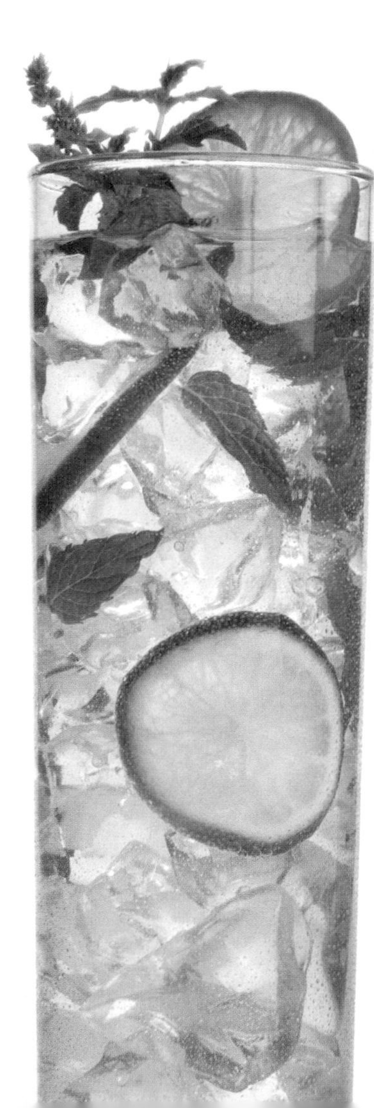

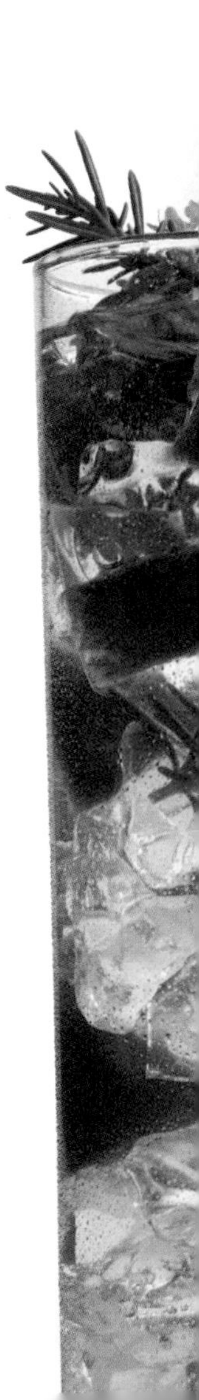

THE BEACHBODY WATER BAR

To help you stay properly hydrated, we've created the Water Bar. Here you can find great ways to make your plain water more interesting.

MIXERS	MIX-INS	
	FRUITS / VEGGIES	HERBS / SPICES
• Flat water • Sparkling water (make sure it has no calories)	• Lemon wedges • Lime wedges • Orange slices • Strawberry slices • Kiwi slices • Mango slices • Pineapple slices • Cucumber slices • Frozen grapes • Watermelon cubes • Honeydew melon cubes • Blueberries • Raspberries • Splash of fruit juice: cranberry, orange, grapefruit	• Mint leaves • Basil • Grated ginger • Rosemary • Tarragon • Cinnamon

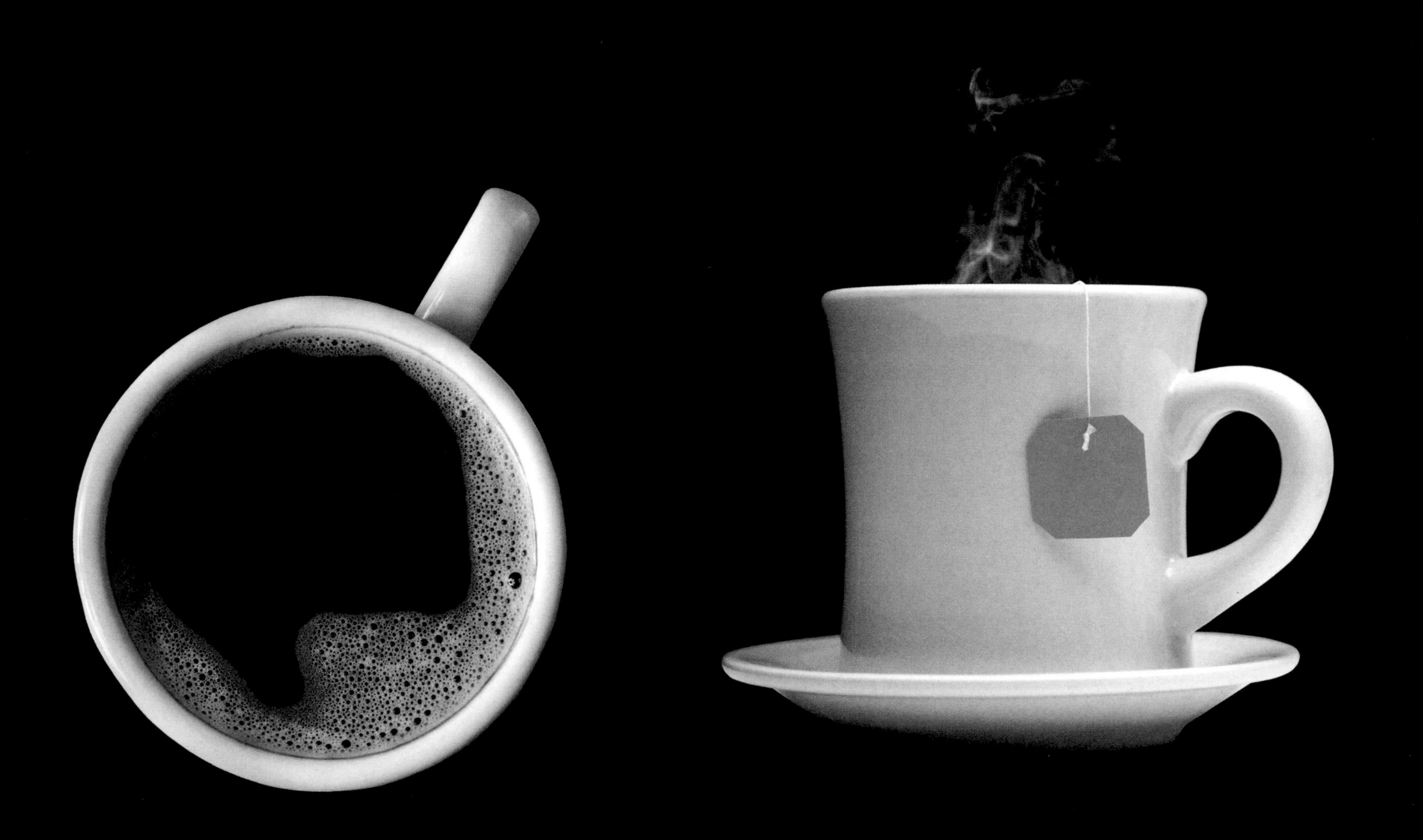

COFFEE AND TEA

Both of these drinks are filled with antioxidants, meaning they can combat the symptoms of stress—and they also have a "slight" fat-burning effect.

Ideally, you'd drink your coffee black and your tea plain. "Tea" by our definition includes decaf, herbal, and UNSWEETENED iced tea. It doesn't include most powdered, canned, and bottled "tea" beverages.

But if you'd like to add a little "something" to your coffee or tea, here are some ideas—and some guidelines as to how much coffee or tea you can drink and some items to stay away from.

UNLIMITED COFFEE OR TEA FLAVOR ADDITIVES:
Cinnamon
Lemon
Pumpkin spice
Nutmeg
Stevia

ONE OR TWO 8-OUNCE CUPS OF COFFEE OR TEA PER DAY WITH THESE FLAVOR ADDITIVES:
1–2 Tablespoons low/nonfat milk
1–2 teaspoons raw sugar, honey, molasses, maple syrup, or agave syrup

STAY AWAY FROM:
Cream
Half-and-half
Nondairy creamer
White (refined) sugar
Artificial sweeteners
Flavored syrups (such as caramel, vanilla, hazelnut, etc.)
Chocolate syrup

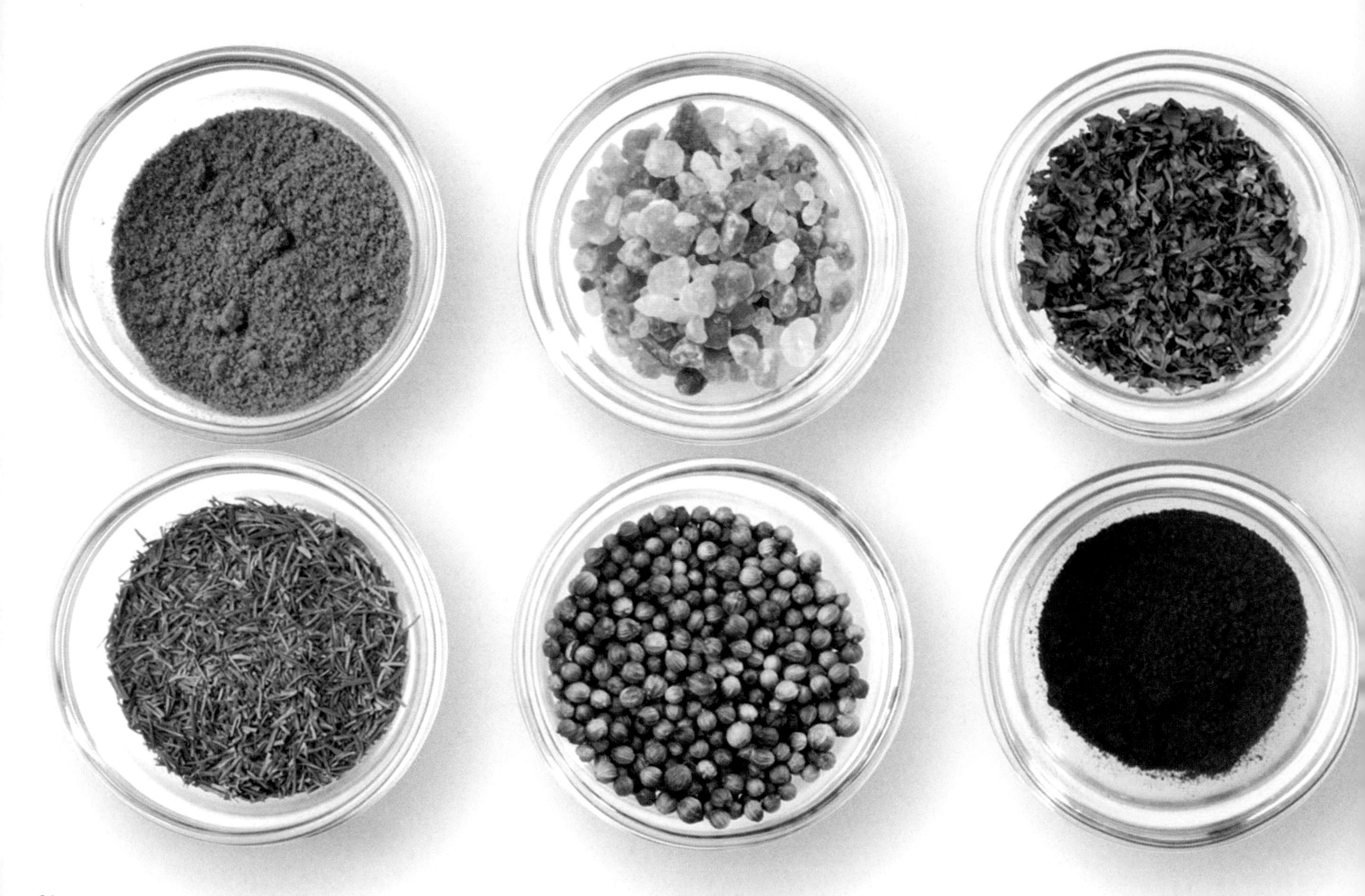

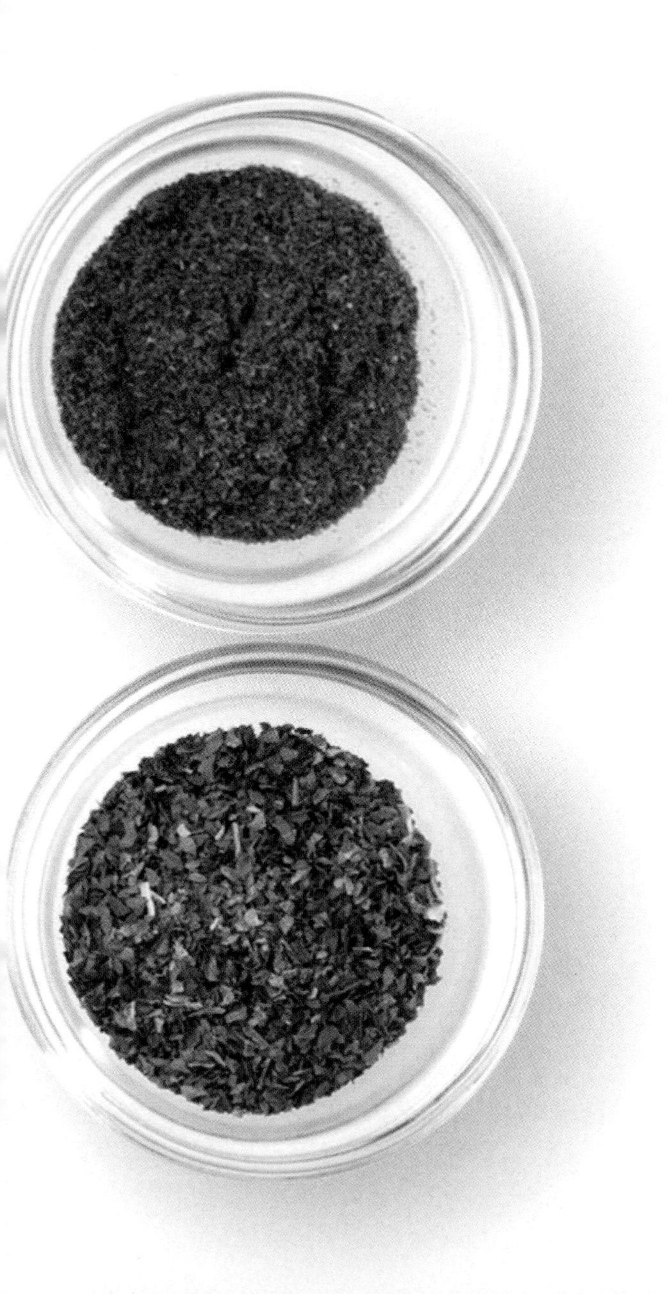

SEASONINGS AND CONDIMENTS

Use as much of these "Free Foods" as you'd like to make your food taste good to you. The calories are fairly inconsequential.

- Lemon and/or lime juice (not lemonade)
- Vinegars (cider, white wine, or red wine)
- Mustard
- Herbs (fresh and dry)
- Spices (except salt)
- Garlic
- Ginger
- Hot sauce (Only Tabasco or Mexican hot sauces that contain little-to-no salt or sugar)
- Flavor extracts (pure vanilla, peppermint, almond, etc.)
- Portion Fix SEASONING MIXES (see pages 42–43)

FAQ

(Frequently Asked Questions)

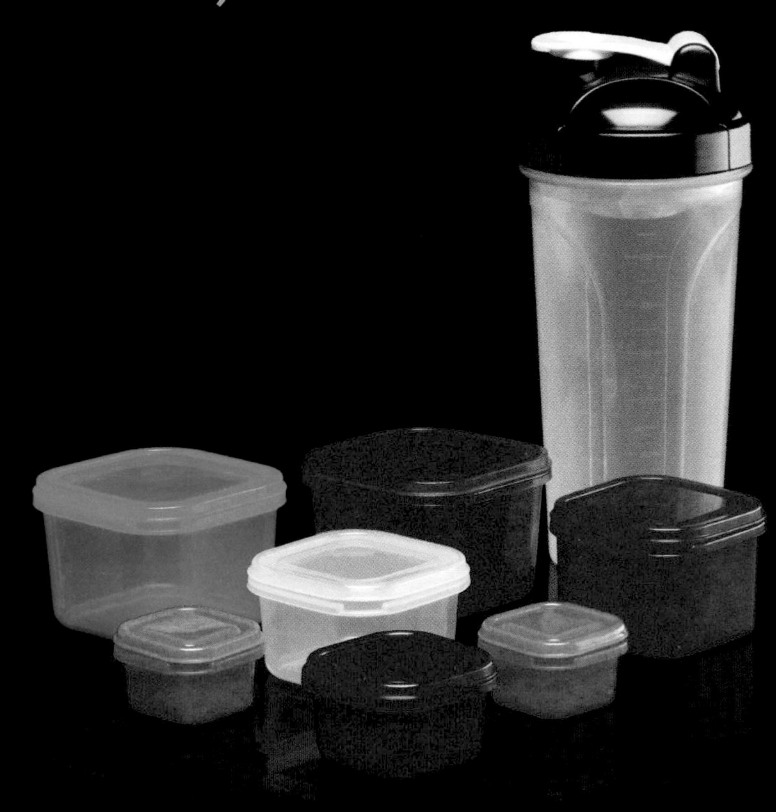

How should I be spacing out my meals? How often should I be eating?

- Spread your meals across the day, eating every 2 to 3 hours (breakfast, lunch, dinner, and one or two snacks). This helps improve nutrient absorption and keeps your energy levels steady.
- Eat breakfast within an hour of waking up. Or if you work out first thing, eat it within 15 minutes of completing your workout to promote recovery.

How do I know when it's time to recalculate my Calorie Target and find a new Portion Plan?

- **If you plateau.** If weight loss (or gain) has stalled, the solution may be as simple as a quick recalculation to get things moving. However, if you're trying to lose weight and this doesn't work, try increasing your calories to the next Portion Plan up. Sometimes, under-eating forces your metabolism to slow so that you can hold onto your emergency fuel supply (body fat). In this situation, increasing calories assures your body it is getting what it needs—and weight loss can resume.
- **If you have a new goal.** When you've lost the weight and want to maintain (or add muscle mass), a quick recalculation should do the trick. To maintain weight, start by recalculating your new Calorie Target on page 7. When you find your Maintenance Calories, stop there. Use that number to find your new Portion Plan. If you want to gain weight or muscle mass, add 350 calories to your Maintenance Calories and use that new Calorie Target to find the correct Portion Plan. (Just make sure to accompany any weight gain goals with serious exercise, otherwise you'll just gain fat, not muscle.)

If you'd like help with your calories, visit the "Expert Advice" section of the Team Beachbody® Message Boards at TeamBeachbody.com. There you can discuss the situation with our knowledgeable, friendly advice staff.

What about my other Beachbody program's nutrition plan?

If you're doing any of Beachbody's other programs, odds are that the nutrition plan might not 100% correspond with the Portion Fix way of eating. That's because the Portion Fix uses a broad nutritional strategy to cover multiple programs.

If you're doing one of our programs, you have two choices. You can stick with the nutrition plan that comes with the program for a more targeted approach. However, the simplicity and ease-of-use that the Portion Fix provides may better suit your needs. You'll get excellent results either way as long as you calculate your caloric needs accurately from the very start.

What if I'm still hungry?

Hunger generally isn't a sign of needing food. It's a sign of being used to a certain amount or type of food. So try your best to overcome it and you should adapt in a week or so. However, if you're having problems sleeping, you're irritable, you're low on energy, or you can't make it through workouts, it's okay to add one of the following to your day: TWO GREENS, ONE PURPLE, ONE BLUE, or ONE ORANGE. But if you're having these issues consistently, you might want to move up to a higher-calorie plan.

RECIPES

Here are a variety of simple, healthy recipes designed and organized according to container to help simplify hitting your color count each day.

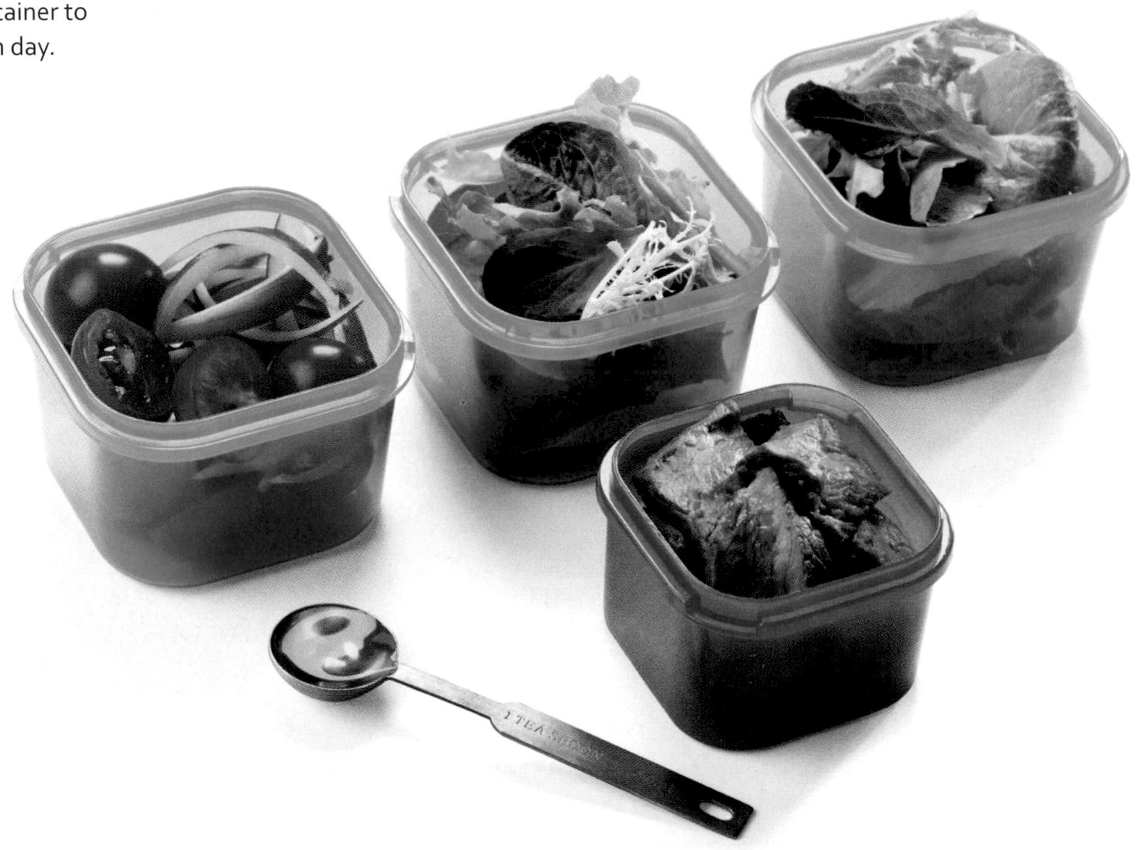

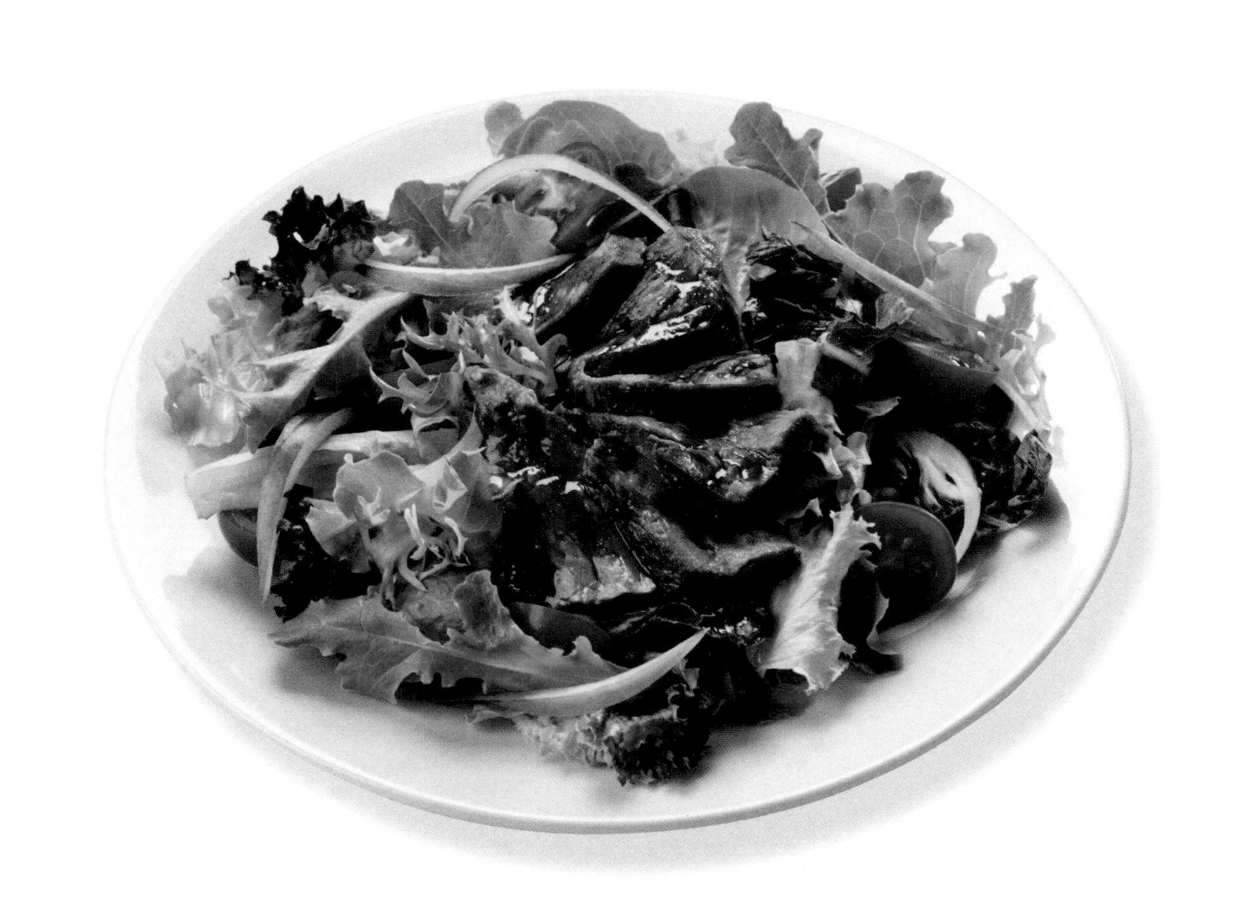

SEASONING MIXES

In addition to the free Seasonings and Condiments on page 37, the seasoning mixes below are also a fast and easy way to bring your savory foods to life without undermining your Portion Plan. Just combine these herbs, mix well, and store them in an airtight container. You can use these mixes as:

- A rub for roasting or grilling chicken, meat, or fish
- A way to spice up ground chicken, turkey, or beef
- A way to flavor rice, lentils, beans, quinoa, and vegetables

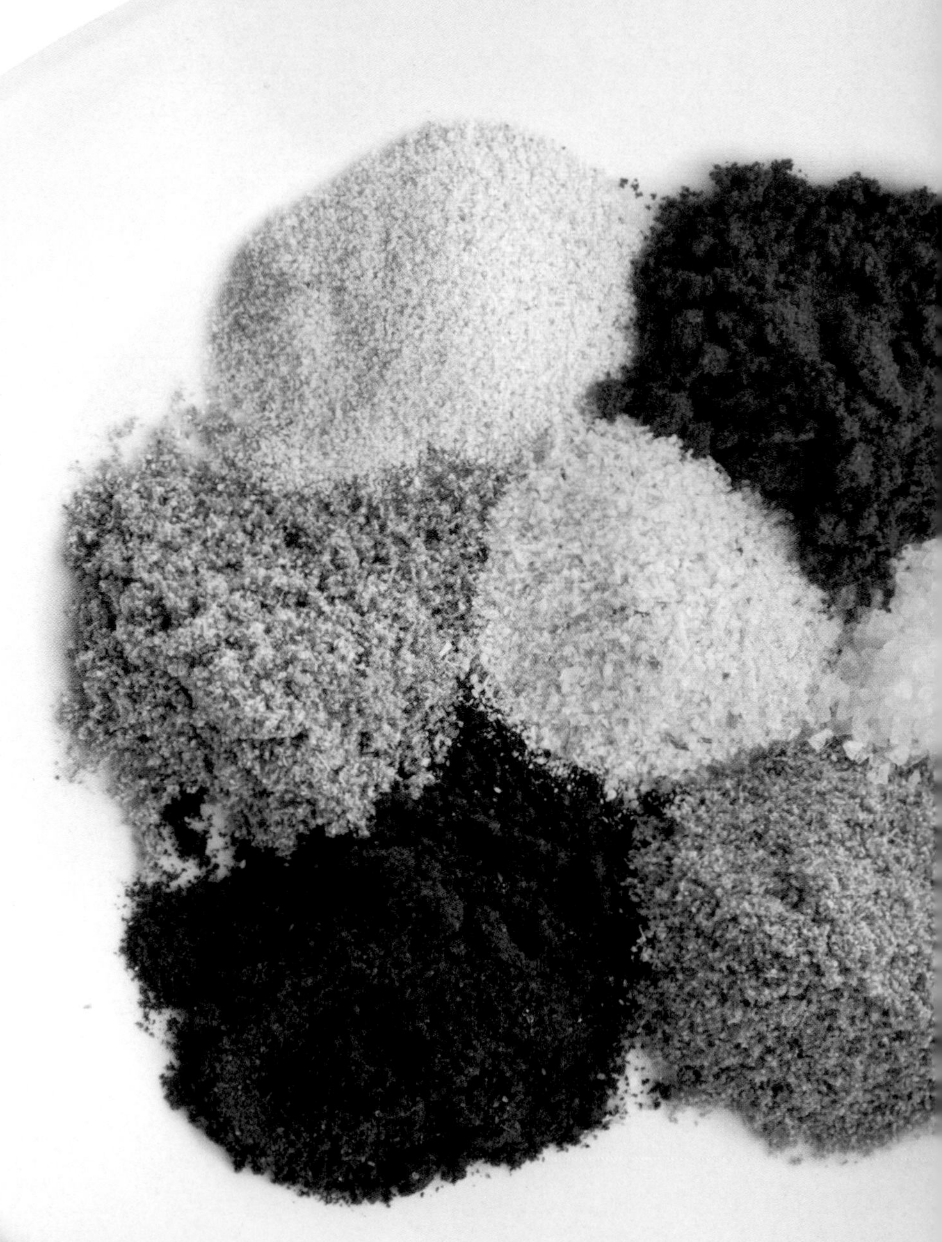

ALL-PURPOSE SEASONING
4 tsp. onion powder
2 tsp. garlic powder
2 tsp. mustard powder
¼ tsp. dried thyme
¼ tsp. ground black pepper
1 tsp. sea salt or Himalayan salt (Mineralize)

SMOKY SOUTHWESTERN SEASONING
1 Tbsp. chili powder
2 tsp. ground cumin
1 tsp. coriander
½ tsp. onion powder
½ tsp. garlic powder
½ tsp. dried oregano
½ tsp. smoked paprika
1 tsp. sea salt or Himalayan salt (Mineralize)

MEDITERRANEAN SEASONING
4 Tbsp. dried parsley, crushed
4 tsp. dried onion flakes
2 tsp. dried basil, crushed
1 tsp. ground oregano
1 tsp. ground thyme
1 tsp. garlic powder
1 tsp. sea salt or Himalayan salt (Mineralize)
¼ tsp. ground black pepper

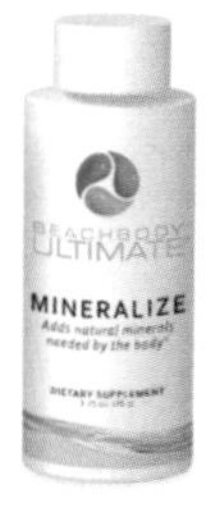

WHY MINERALIZE?

Nourish your body with our natural Himalayan salt, containing up to 84 essential, naturally occurring minerals and trace elements. Helps aid in nutrient absorption and supports nervous system function.*

Minerals, including salt, are essential to life. Our Mineralize contains pure natural Himalayan crystal salt, minimally processed and containing up to 84 naturally occurring minerals and trace elements, such as calcium, magnesium, potassium, copper, and iron.

Natural salt replaces the essential minerals which are vital to life, from building strong bones to nervous system function, aiding in the absorption of nutrients through the digestive tract, and even helping to prevent muscle cramps.*

TO LEARN MORE, CONTACT YOUR TEAM BEACHBODY COACH OR GO TO BUYMINERALIZE.COM

*These statements have not been evaluated by the Food and Drug Administration. This product is not intended to diagnose, treat, cure, or prevent any disease.

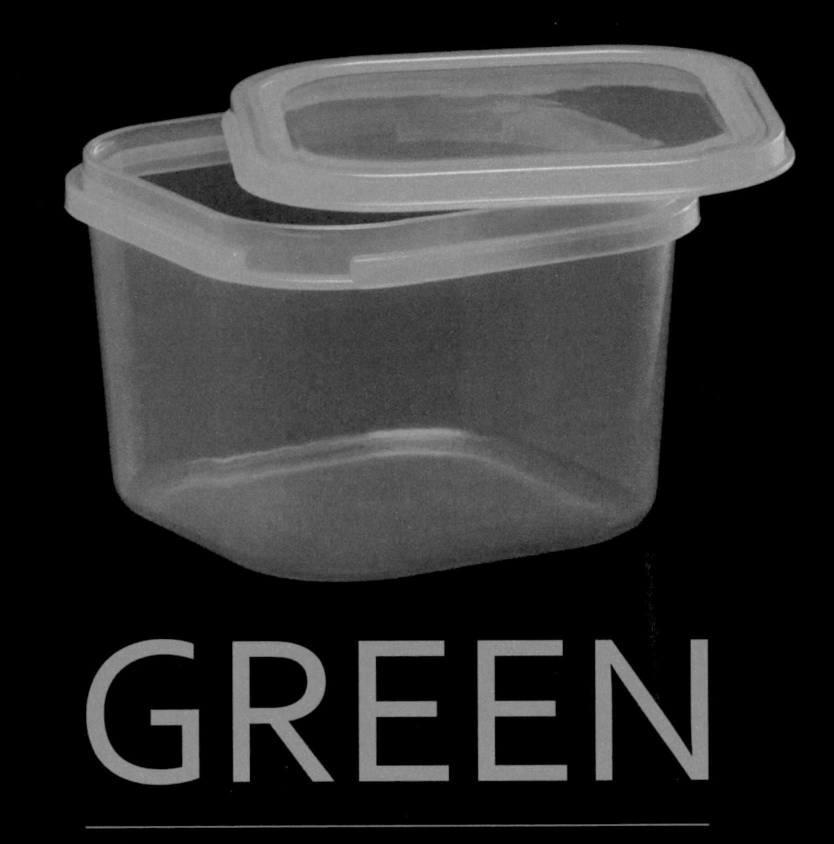

GREEN

[NOTE: All Green Container recipes count for one Green Container portion and one teaspoon portion.]

SAUTÉED KALE

(Makes 1 serving)

Container Equivalents (per serving):
One Green Container and
One Teaspoon

1 tsp.	olive oil
¼ cup	chopped onion
2 cups	chopped raw kale
½ tsp.	All-Purpose Seasoning or Mediterranean Seasoning (see pg. 42)

1. Heat oil in medium skillet over medium heat.
2. Cook onion, stirring frequently for 2 minutes or until translucent.
3. Add kale and Seasoning; continue cooking for 3 to 5 minutes or until kale is wilted.

MIXED VEGGIE STIR-FRY

(Makes 1 serving)

Container Equivalents (per serving):
One Green Container and
One Teaspoon

1 tsp.	olive oil
¼ cup	chopped asparagus spears
¼ cup	chopped red bell pepper
¼ cup	chopped carrots
¼ cup	chopped onions
½ tsp.	Mediterranean Seasoning or All-Purpose Seasoning (see pg. 42)

1. Heat oil in medium skillet over medium heat.
2. Combine asparagus, pepper, carrots, onions, and Seasoning.
3. Cook vegetables in skillet, mixing frequently for 2 to 3 minutes or until tender-crisp.

COOKING TIP:
Add finely chopped fresh ginger from the SEASONINGS AND CONDIMENTS list to add additional flavor to your veggies.

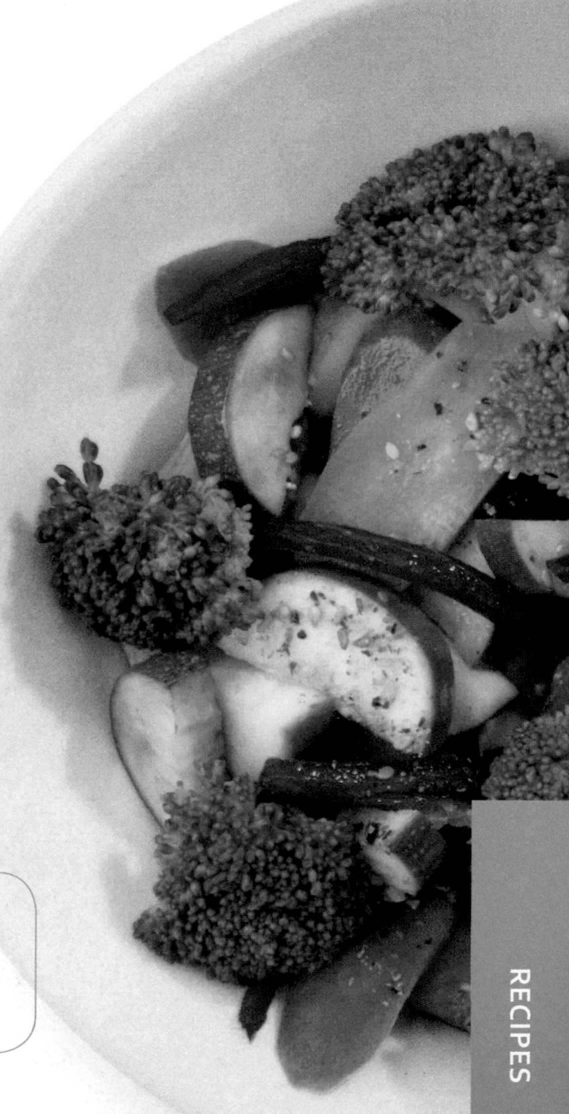

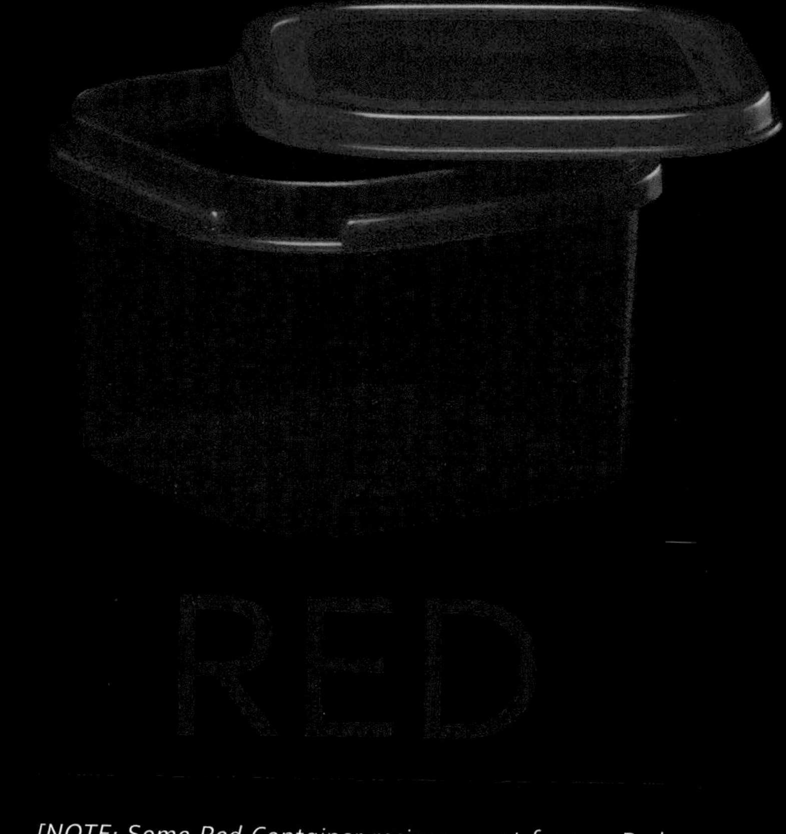

[NOTE: Some Red Container recipes count for one Red Container portion and One Teaspoon portion. Others are just one Red Container, so pay attention.]

HARD-BOILED EGGS

(Makes 1 serving, 2 eggs each)

Container Equivalents (per serving):
■ One Red Container

2 large eggs
Cold water

1. Place eggs in saucepan and add cold water to cover eggs by one inch.
2. Bring water just to a boil over high heat. Remove from heat, cover, and let stand for 12 minutes.
3. Remove from hot water and serve warm or rinse in cold water until cool.

SCRAMBLED EGGS

(Makes 1 serving, 2 eggs each)

Container Equivalents (per serving):
■ One Red Container

Nonstick cooking spray
2 large eggs, lightly beaten

1. Heat nonstick skillet lightly coated with spray over medium-low heat. Add eggs; cook, stirring occasionally, for 3 to 5 minutes, or until eggs are set.

POACHED EGGS

(Makes 1 serving, 2 eggs each)

Container Equivalents (per serving):
■ One Red Container

1 cup water
½ tsp. fresh lemon juice (or white vinegar)
2 large eggs

1. Place water in medium saucepan and bring to a boil over medium-high heat. Add lemon juice; reduce heat to maintain a gentle boil.
2. Break eggs into a small bowl. Hold bowl close to the water's surface and slip the eggs, one by one, into the water. Cook until whites are completely set and yolks begin to thicken, about 5 minutes. Gently lift eggs out of water; keep warm.

SERVING TIP:
Sprinkle eggs with Smoky Southwestern Seasoning (see pg. 42).

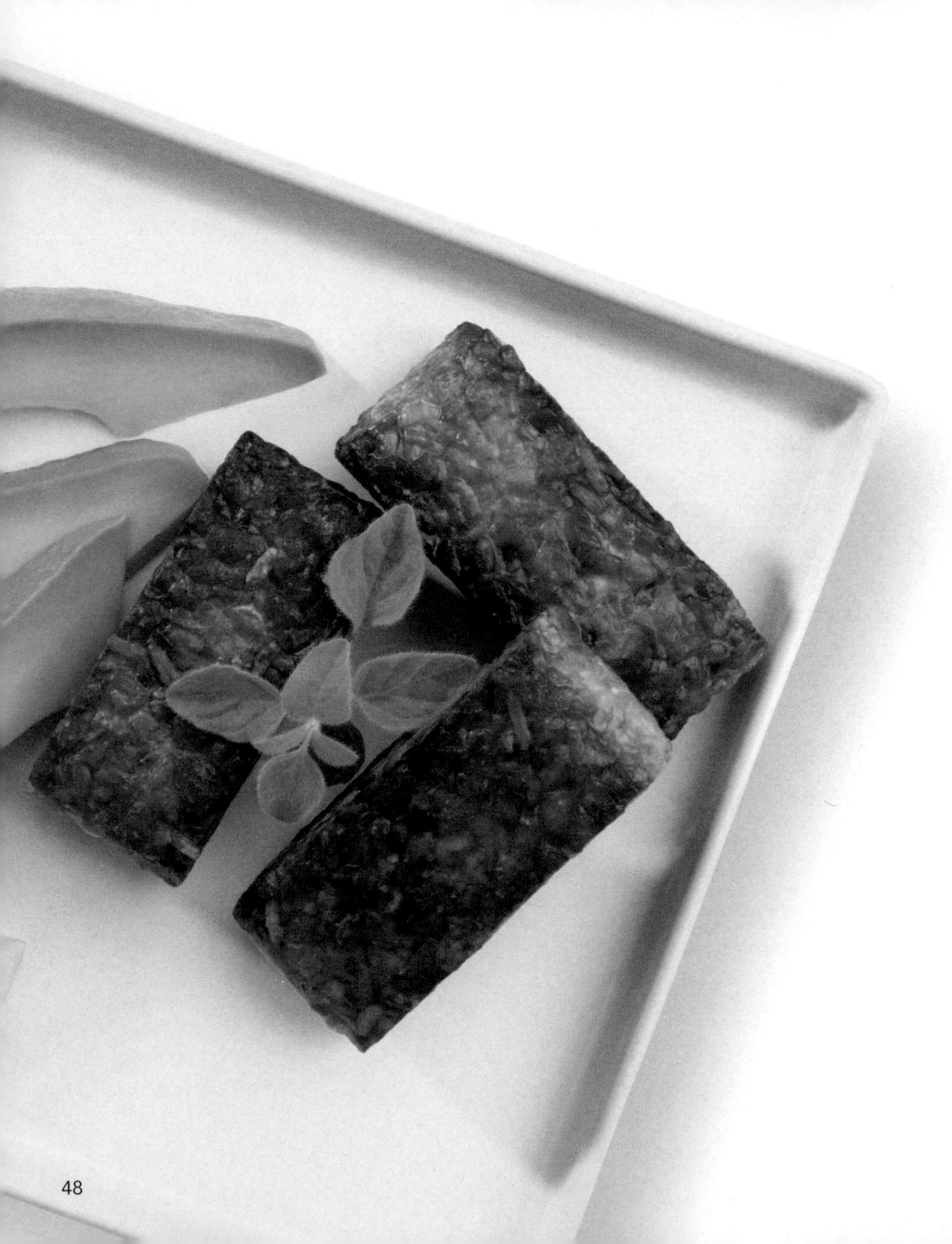

CUMIN TEMPEH STRIPS

(Makes 1 serving)

Container Equivalents (per serving):
One Red Container and
One Teaspoon

5 oz	soy tempeh
1 tsp.	olive oil
1 dash	ground cumin
1 dash	smoked paprika
	Sea salt or Himalayan salt (Mineralize) to taste

1. Cut tempeh into strips; drizzle both sides evenly with oil.
2. Season both sides of tempeh strips evenly with salt, cumin, and paprika.
3. Heat medium skillet over medium heat. Cook tempeh for 2 to 3 minutes on both sides.

BAKED CHICKEN BREAST

(Makes 1 serving)

Container Equivalents (per serving):
One Red Container and
One Teaspoon

4 oz	raw chicken breast, boneless, skinless
1 tsp.	olive oil
	All-Purpose Seasoning or Smoky Southwestern Seasoning (see pg. 42) (to taste; optional)

1. Preheat oven to 375° F.
2. Place chicken in ovenproof dish.
3. Drizzle with oil. Season with All-Purpose Seasoning or Smoky Southwestern Seasoning (if desired).
4. Bake for 15 to 20 minutes or until chicken is no longer pink in the middle and juices run clear.

COOKING TIP:
Cooking times may vary depending on the thickness and weight of the chicken breasts. Cook chicken breast for the following times:
3 to 6 oz – 15 to 20 minutes
7 to 12 oz – 18 to 25 minutes
13 to 16 oz – 20 to 30 minutes
You can also season chicken with lemon or lime juice and dry herbs like rosemary and thyme.

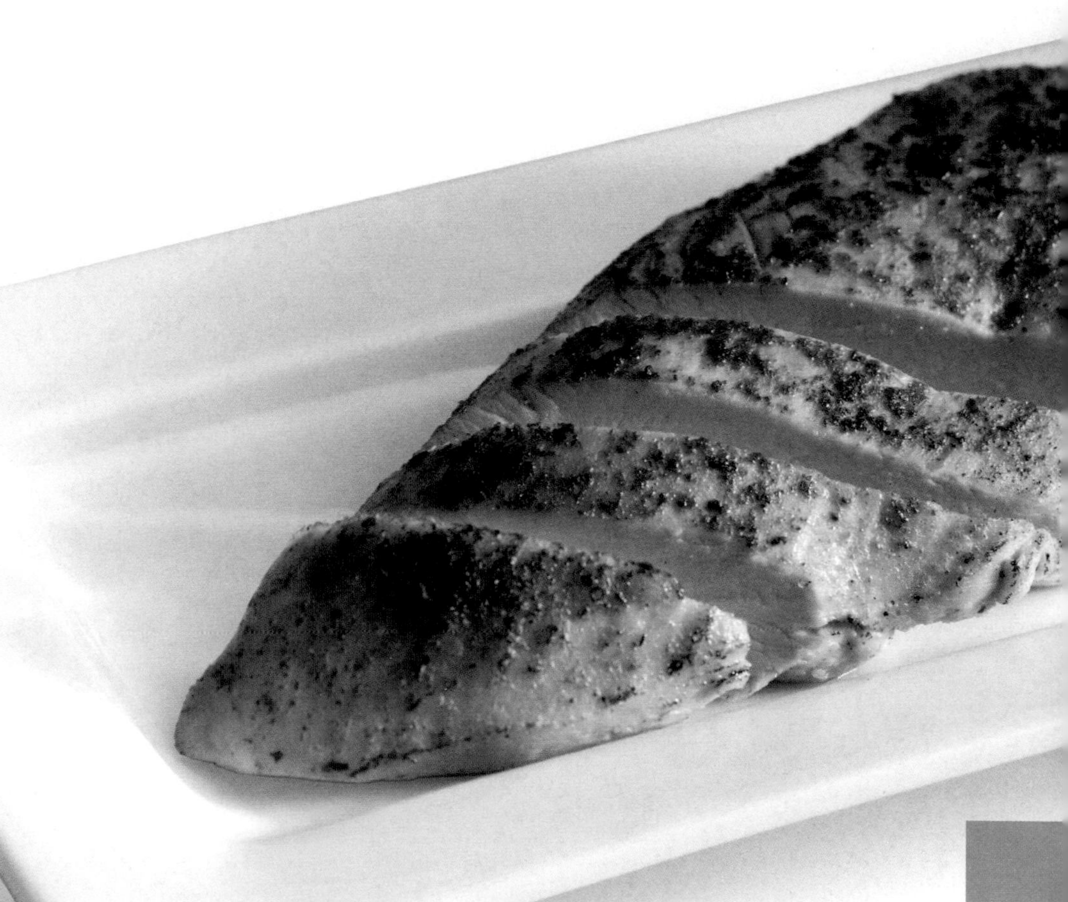

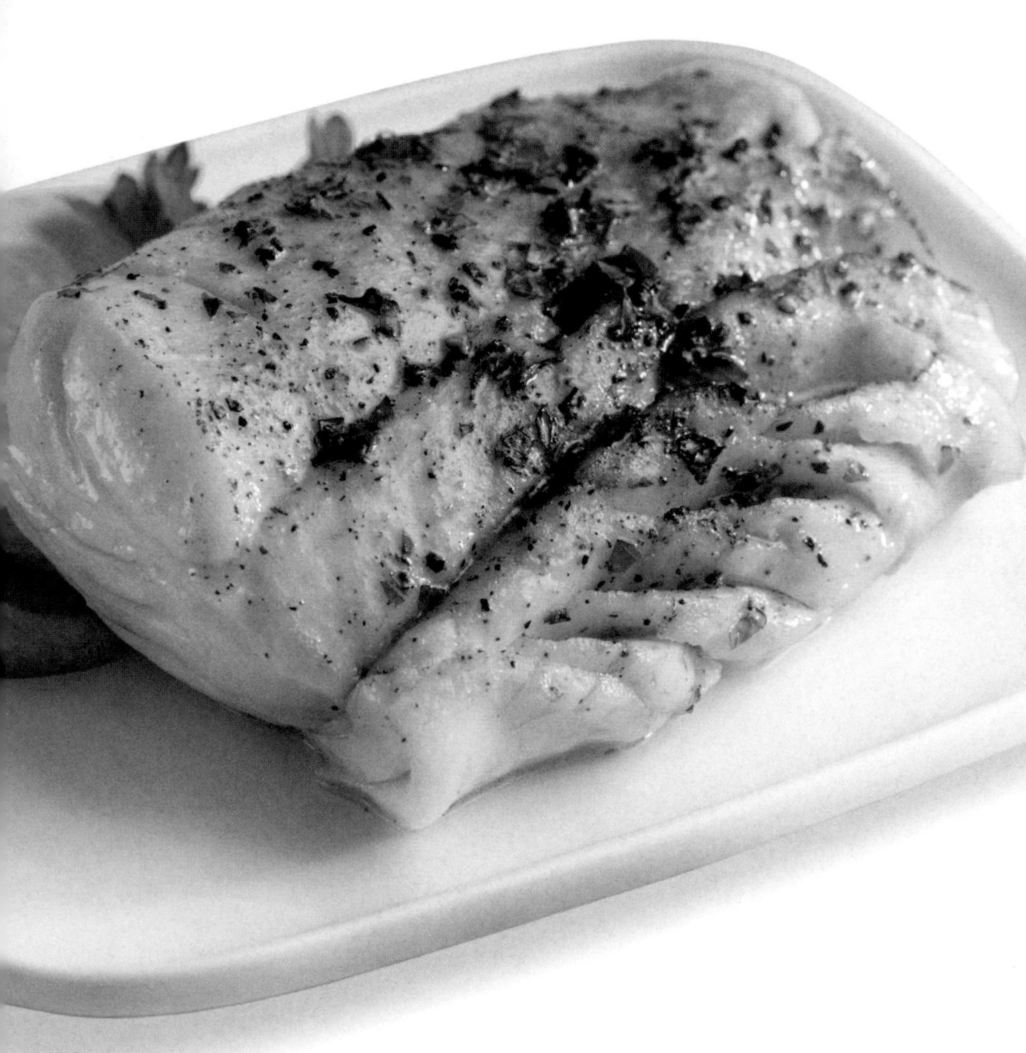

WHITE FISH

(Makes 1 serving)

Container Equivalents (per serving):
One Red Container and
One Teaspoon

4 oz	raw white fish (such as cod, tilapia, halibut, etc.)
1 tsp.	olive oil
	All-Purpose Seasoning or Mediterranean Seasoning (see pg. 42) (to taste; optional)

1. Preheat broiler to high.
2. Drizzle with oil. Season with All-Purpose Seasoning or Mediterranean Seasoning (if desired).
3. Broil fish for about 3 to 4 minutes on each side or until fish is opaque and flakes easily when tested with a fork.

COOKING TIP:
Cooking times may vary depending on the thickness and weight of the fish. Cook fish for the following times:
4 to 6 oz – 5 to 7 minutes on each side
7 to 12 oz – 6 to 9 minutes on each side
13 to 16 oz – 7 to 10 minutes on each side
You can also season fish with lemon or lime juice and dry herbs like dill and basil.

BEEF

(Makes 1 serving)

Container Equivalents (per serving):
One Red Container and
One Teaspoon

4 oz	raw beef (such as flank steak, beef sirloin, beef tri-tip, etc.)
1 tsp.	olive oil
	All-Purpose Seasoning or Smoky Southwestern Seasoning (see pg. 42) (to taste; optional)

1. Preheat grill or broiler to high.
2. Drizzle with oil. Season with All-Purpose Seasoning or Smoky Southwestern Seasoning (if desired).
3. Grill or broil beef for about 4 to 5 minutes on each side for medium-rare, or 6 to 7 minutes on each side for medium. Remove from heat; let stand for 5 minutes.

COOKING TIP:
Cooking times may vary depending on the thickness and weight of the beef. For medium-rare, cook beef for the following times:
3 to 6 oz – 4 to 7 minutes on each side
7 to 12 oz – 6 to 9 minutes on each side
13 to 16 oz – 7 to 10 minutes on each side
You can also season beef with garlic and dry herbs like sage and parsley.

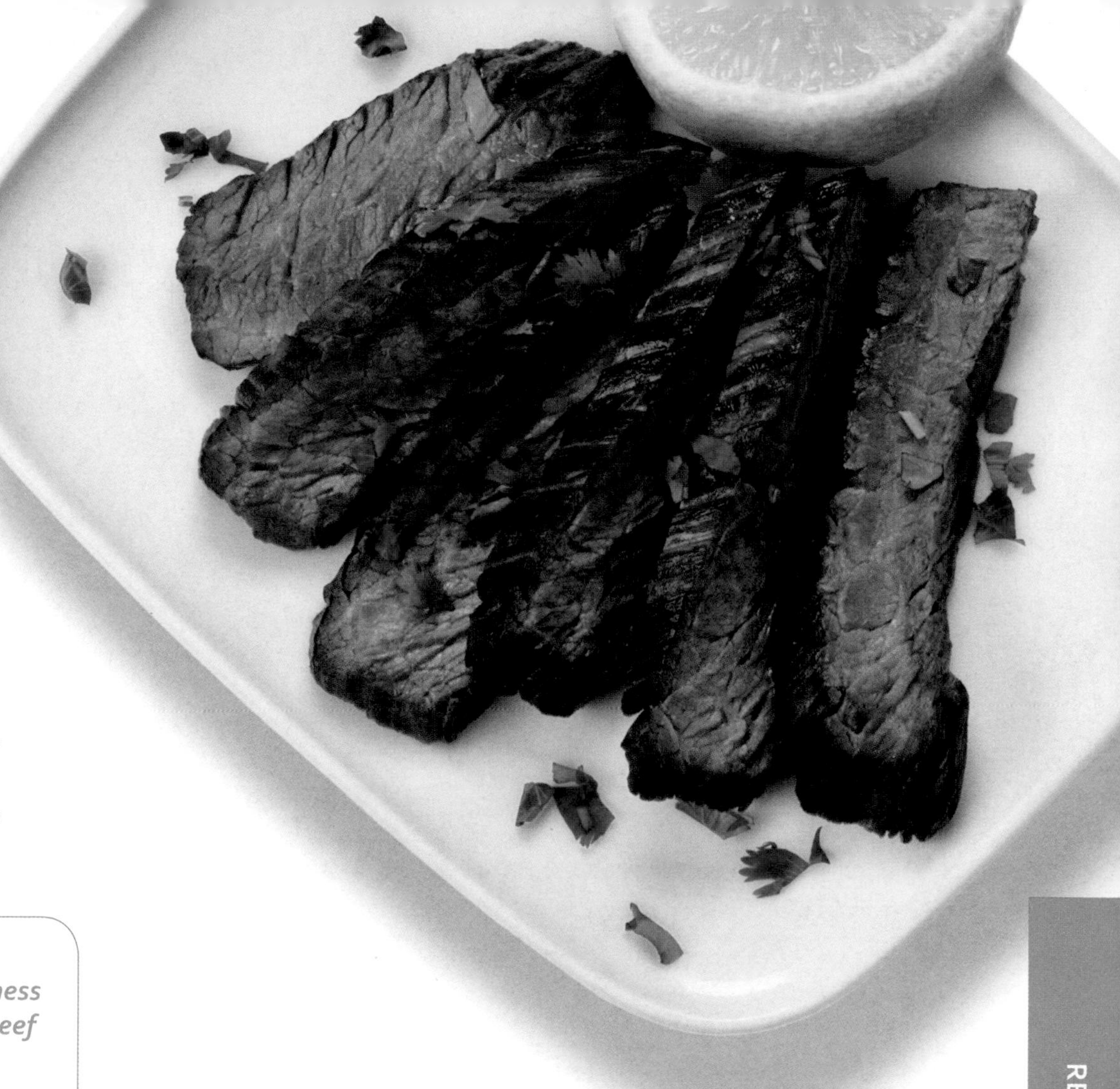

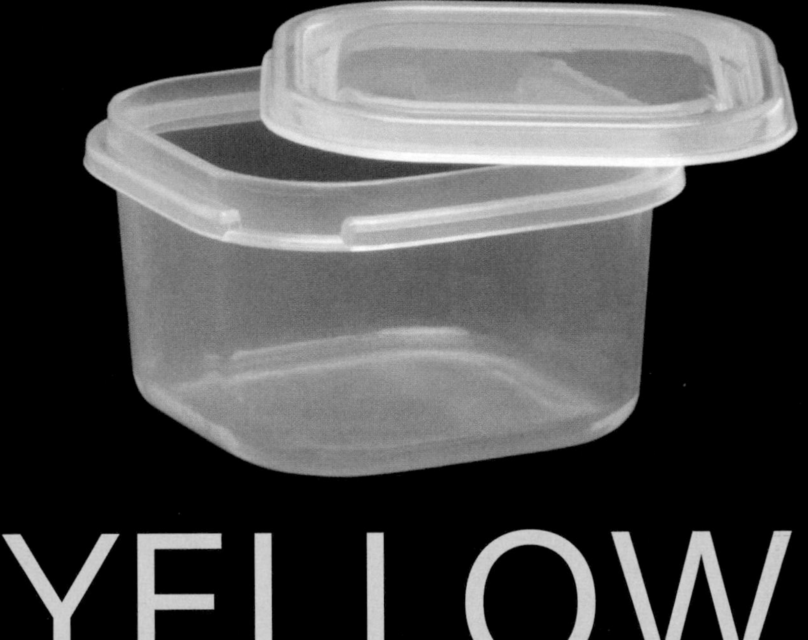

YELLOW

[NOTE: All Yellow Container recipes count for one Yellow Container portion.]

BROWN RICE

(Makes 4 servings)

Container Equivalents (per serving):
One Yellow Container

1 cup	dry brown rice
2 cups	cold water
	Sea salt or Himalayan salt (Mineralize) and ground black pepper (to taste; optional)

1. Combine rice, water, salt (if desired), and pepper (if desired) in medium saucepan and bring to a boil over high heat.
2. Reduce heat to maintain a gentle boil; cook, covered, for 50 minutes. Keep covered the entire time or rice will not cook evenly.
3. Remove pan from heat and let rice rest, covered, for 10 minutes. Do not remove lid.
4. Fluff with a fork and serve.

COOKING TIP:
As a convenience, you can cook more rice than you need and store the leftovers in the refrigerator for up to 4 days. For Spanish-style rice, skip the optional sea salt and pepper and use the Smoky Southwestern Seasoning (see pg. 42) after it's cooked.

Add chopped fresh herbs from the SEASONINGS AND CONDIMENTS list (see pg. 37) to add flavor and color to your rice.

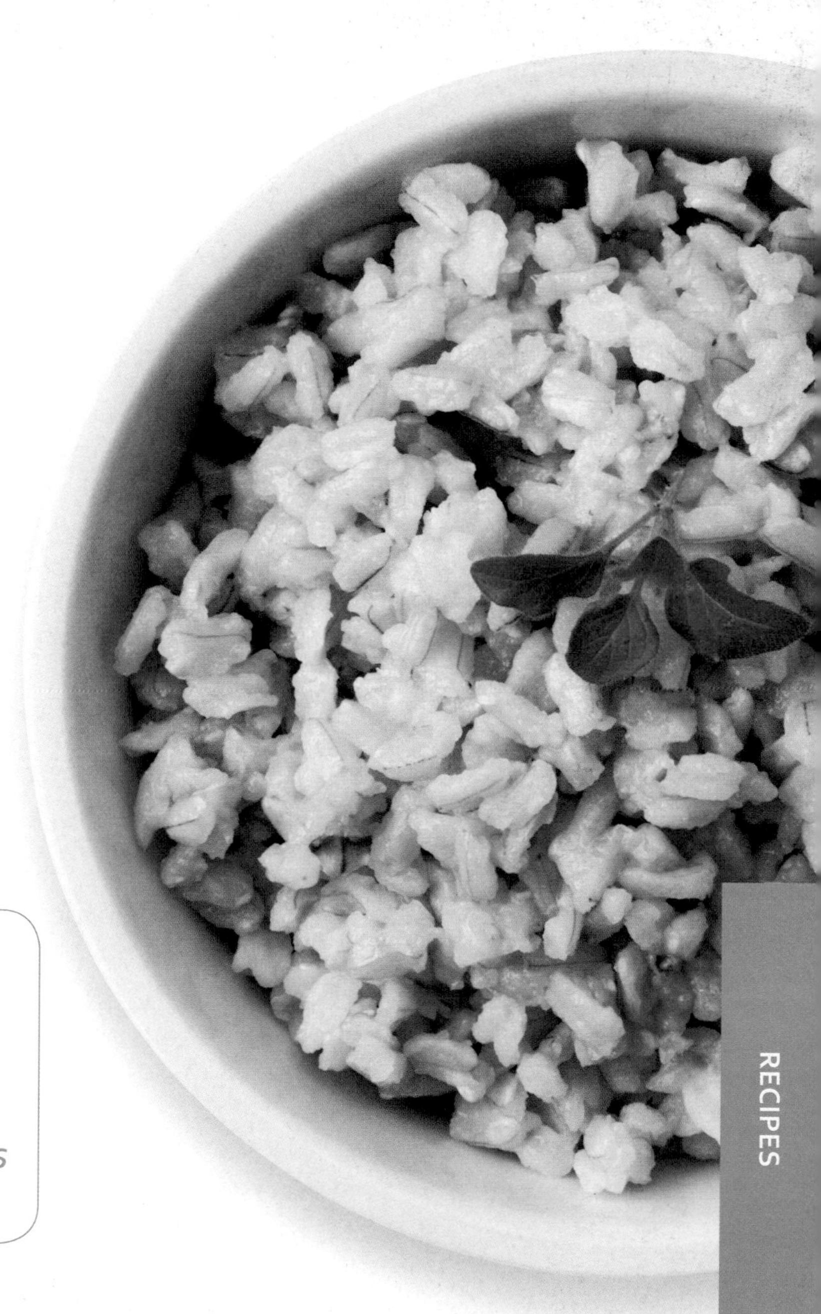

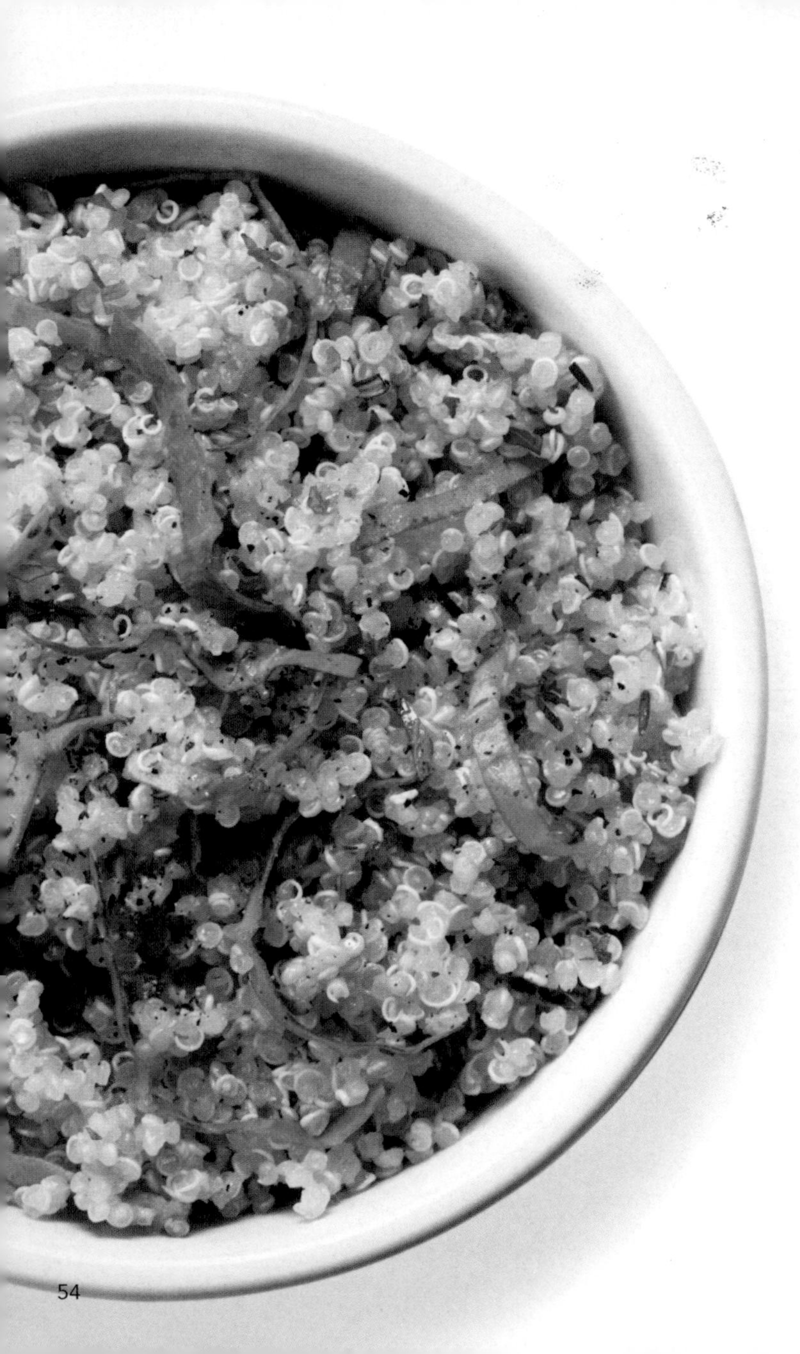

QUINOA

(Makes 4 servings)

Container Equivalents (per serving):
One Yellow Container

1 cup	dry quinoa
2 cups	cold water
	Sea salt or Himalayan salt (Mineralize) and ground black pepper (to taste; optional)

1. Rinse quinoa thoroughly.
2. Combine quinoa, water, salt (if desired), and pepper (if desired) in medium saucepan and bring to a boil over high heat.
3. Reduce heat to maintain a gentle boil; cook, covered, for 15 minutes or until all water has been absorbed.
4. Remove pan from heat and let quinoa rest, covered, for 5 minutes.
5. Fluff with a fork and serve.

COOKING TIP:
As a convenience, you can cook more quinoa than you need and store the leftovers in the refrigerator for up to 4 days. For flavored quinoa, skip the optional sea salt and pepper and use the All-Purpose Seasoning (see pg. 42) after it's cooked.

Add chopped fresh herbs from the SEASONINGS AND CONDIMENTS list (see pg. 37) to add flavor and color to your quinoa.

LENTILS

(Makes 6 servings)

Container Equivalents (per serving):
One Yellow Container

1 cup	dry brown lentils
1¾ cups	water
	Sea salt or Himalayan salt (Mineralize) and ground black pepper (to taste; optional)

1. Sort through the lentils to make sure there are no small stones. Rinse lentils in colander under cool water.
2. Bring water, salt (if desired), and pepper (if desired) to a boil in a medium saucepan over high heat; add lentils.
3. Bring back to a boil; cover, and reduce heat to maintain a gentle boil. Cook for 20 minutes or until lentils are tender.

COOKING TIP:
As a convenience, you can cook more lentils than you need and store the leftovers in the refrigerator for up to 4 days. For flavored lentils, skip the optional sea salt and pepper and use the All-Purpose Seasoning or Smoky Southwestern Seasoning (see pg. 42) after they're cooked.

Add chopped fresh herbs from the SEASONINGS AND CONDIMENTS list (see pg. 37) to add flavor and color to your lentils.

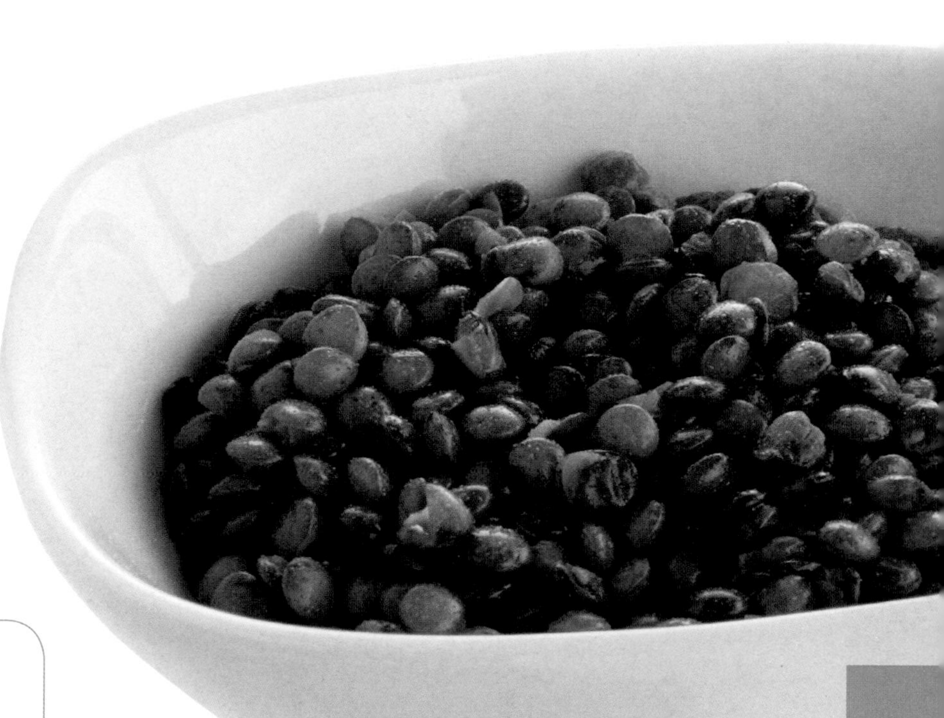

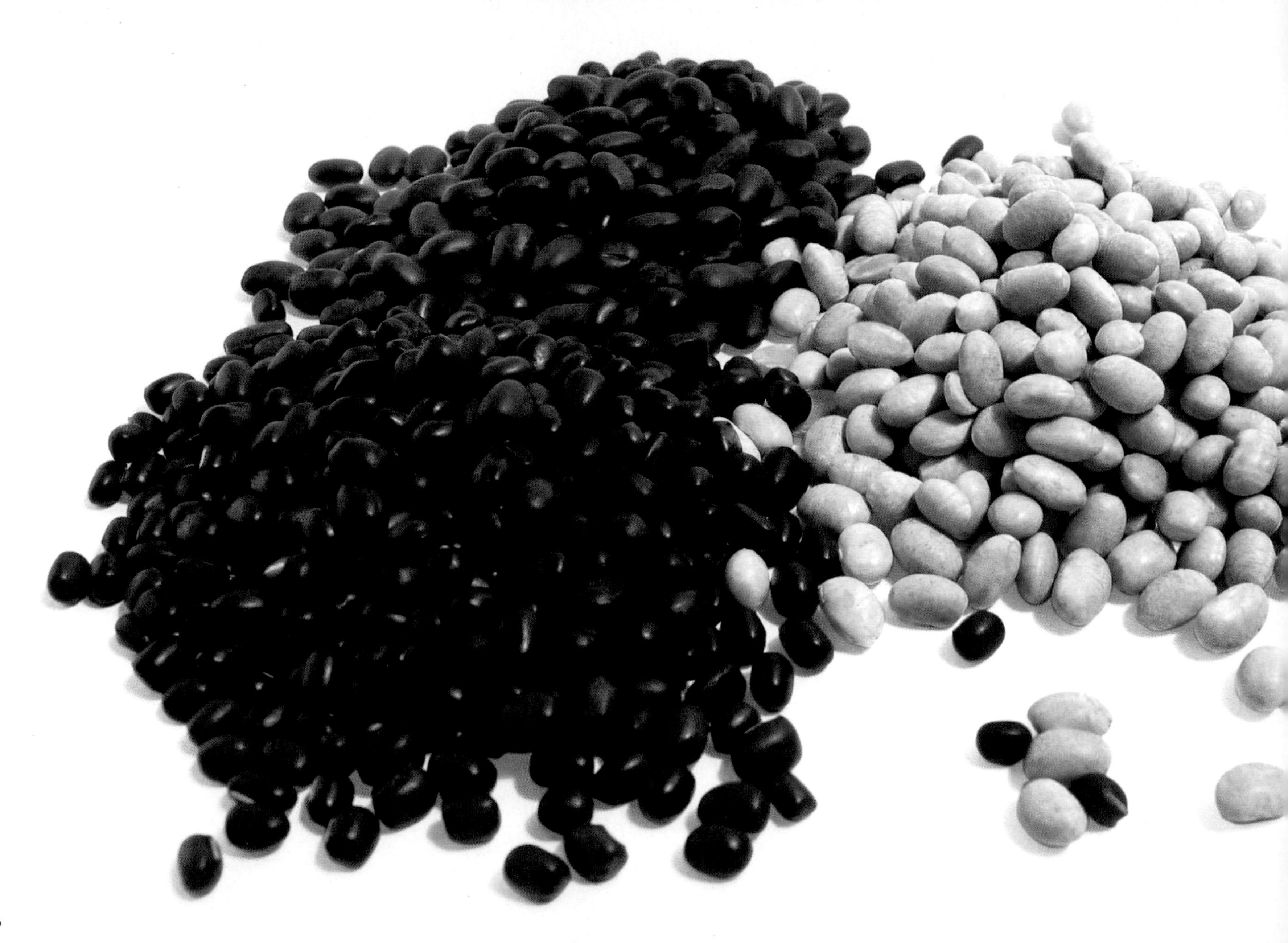

BEANS

(Makes 6 servings)

Container Equivalents (per serving):
One Yellow Container

1 cup	dry beans
3 cups	water
	Sea salt or Himalayan salt (Mineralize) and ground black pepper (to taste; optional)

1. Rinse beans in colander under cool water.
2. Place beans and water in medium saucepan. Soak for 6 hours or preferably overnight. Drain; discard water.
3. Place beans in large saucepan; add water to cover beans by two inches and salt (if desired) and pepper (if desired). Bring to a boil over high heat. Cover, and reduce heat to maintain a gentle boil; cook for 60 to 90 minutes or until beans are tender.

COOKING TIP:
As a convenience, you can cook more beans than you need and store the leftovers in the refrigerator for up to 4 days. For flavored beans, skip the optional sea salt and pepper and use the All-Purpose Seasoning or Smoky Southwestern Seasoning (see pg. 42) after they're cooked.

Add chopped fresh herbs from the SEASONINGS AND CONDIMENTS list (see pg. 37) to add flavor and color to your beans.

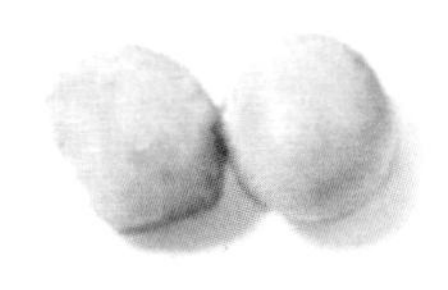

DRESSINGS

These delicious and savory dressings will make your salads come to life.

Just pour any of these dressings into an orange container to measure out one serving.

[NOTE: One serving of each of these dressings satisfies one Orange Container portion.]

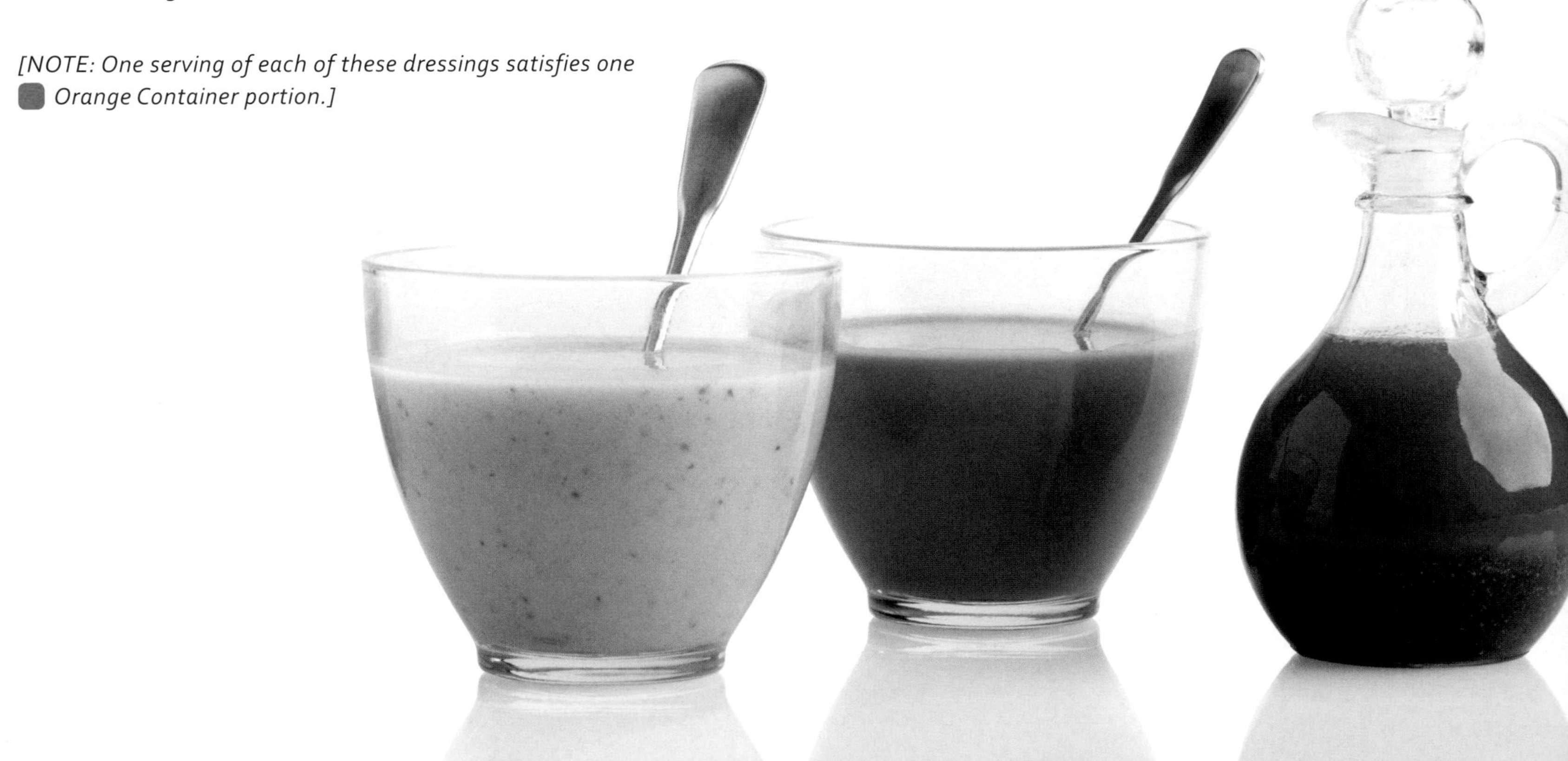

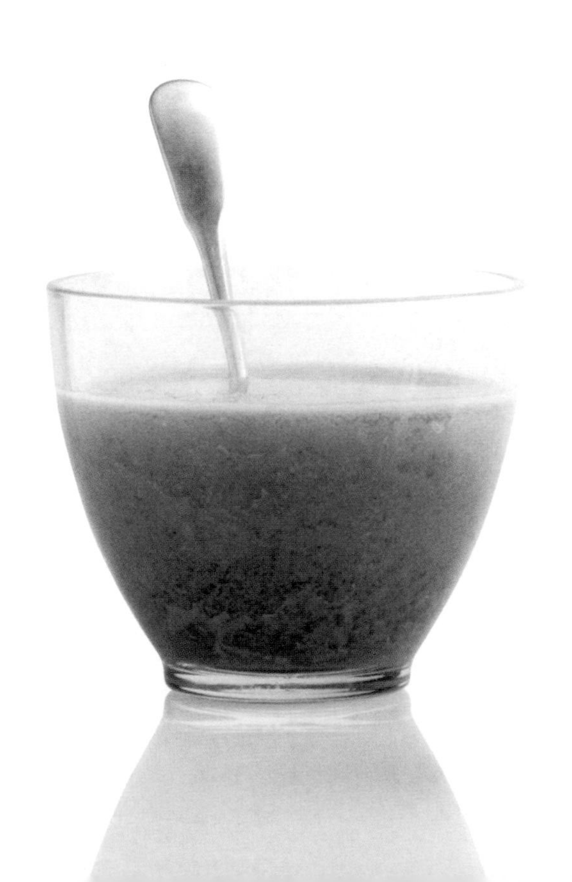

BALSAMIC VINAIGRETTE

(Makes 8 servings, about 2 Tbsp. each)

Container Equivalents (per serving):
One Orange Container

6 Tbsp.	balsamic vinegar
¼ cup	fresh lemon juice
1 tsp.	raw honey (or pure maple syrup)
2 tsp.	Dijon mustard
6 Tbsp.	extra-virgin olive oil

1. Combine vinegar, lemon juice, and honey in a medium bowl; whisk to blend.
2. Stir in mustard; mix well.
3. Slowly add oil while whisking; mix well.

TIP/SERVING SUGGESTION:
Store leftover dressing in a covered container in the refrigerator. If dressing thickens when cold, hold at room temperature for 30 minutes and stir before serving.

This dressing is wonderful on salads, but also great drizzled over sautéed veggies, steamed fish, or grilled chicken and beef.

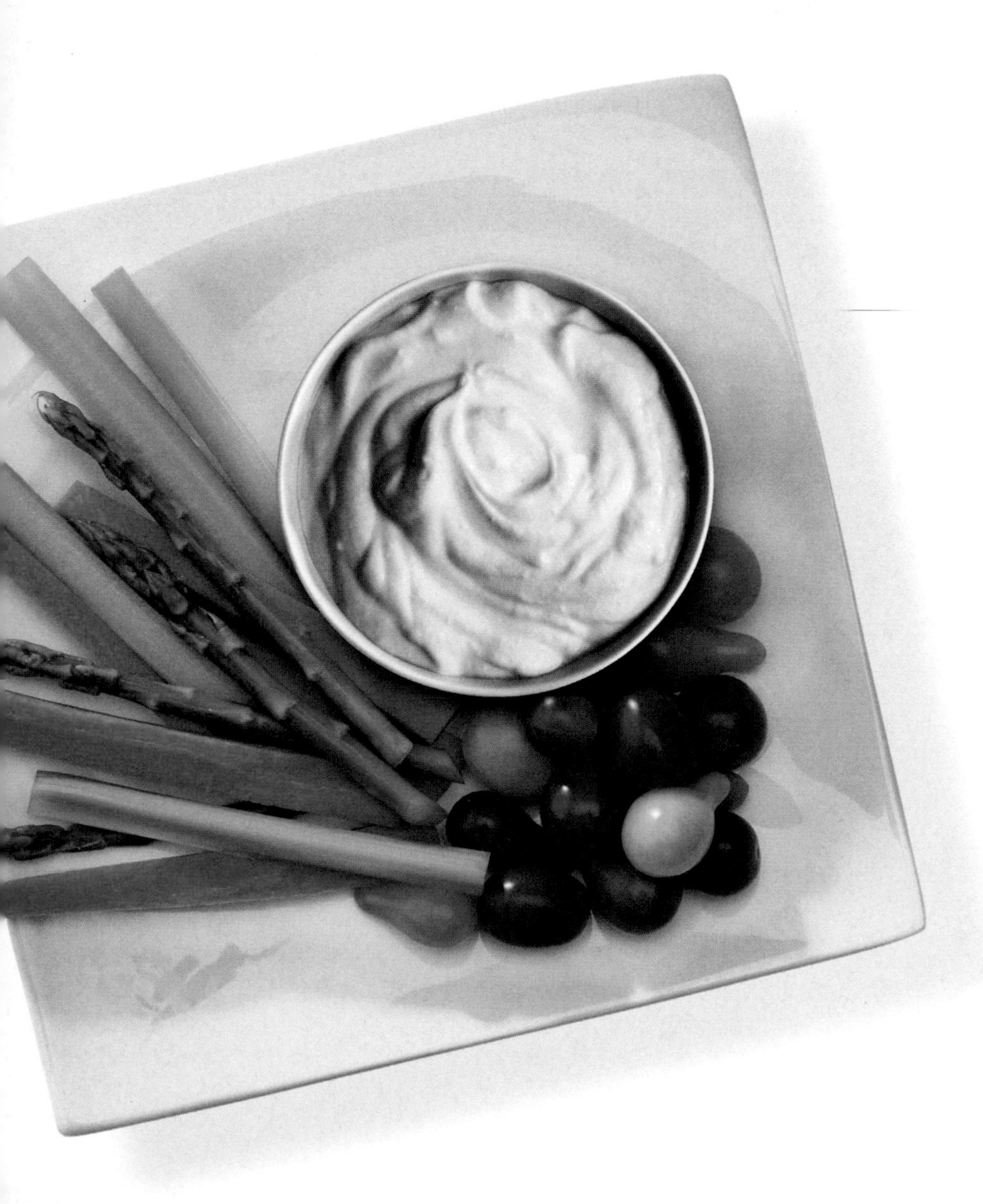

CREAMY HERB DRESSING

(Makes 12 servings, about 2 Tbsp. each)

Container Equivalents (per serving):
■ One Orange Container

1	medium avocado, cut into chunks
1½ cups	nonfat plain Greek yogurt
4 Tbsp.	finely chopped herbs (like tarragon, parsley, mint, or cilantro)
3 Tbsp.	fresh lemon juice
¼ tsp.	sea salt or Himalayan salt (Mineralize)
1 dash	ground white pepper
⅓ cup	extra-virgin olive oil

1. Place avocado, yogurt, herbs, lemon juice, salt, and pepper in a blender; cover. Blend until smooth.
2. Continue blending avocado mixture, slowly adding oil until well blended.
3. Store in the refrigerator, tightly covered, until ready for use.

TIP/SERVING SUGGESTION:
Store leftover dressing in a covered container in the refrigerator.

This dressing is wonderful on salads, but also great as a dip for raw vegetables.

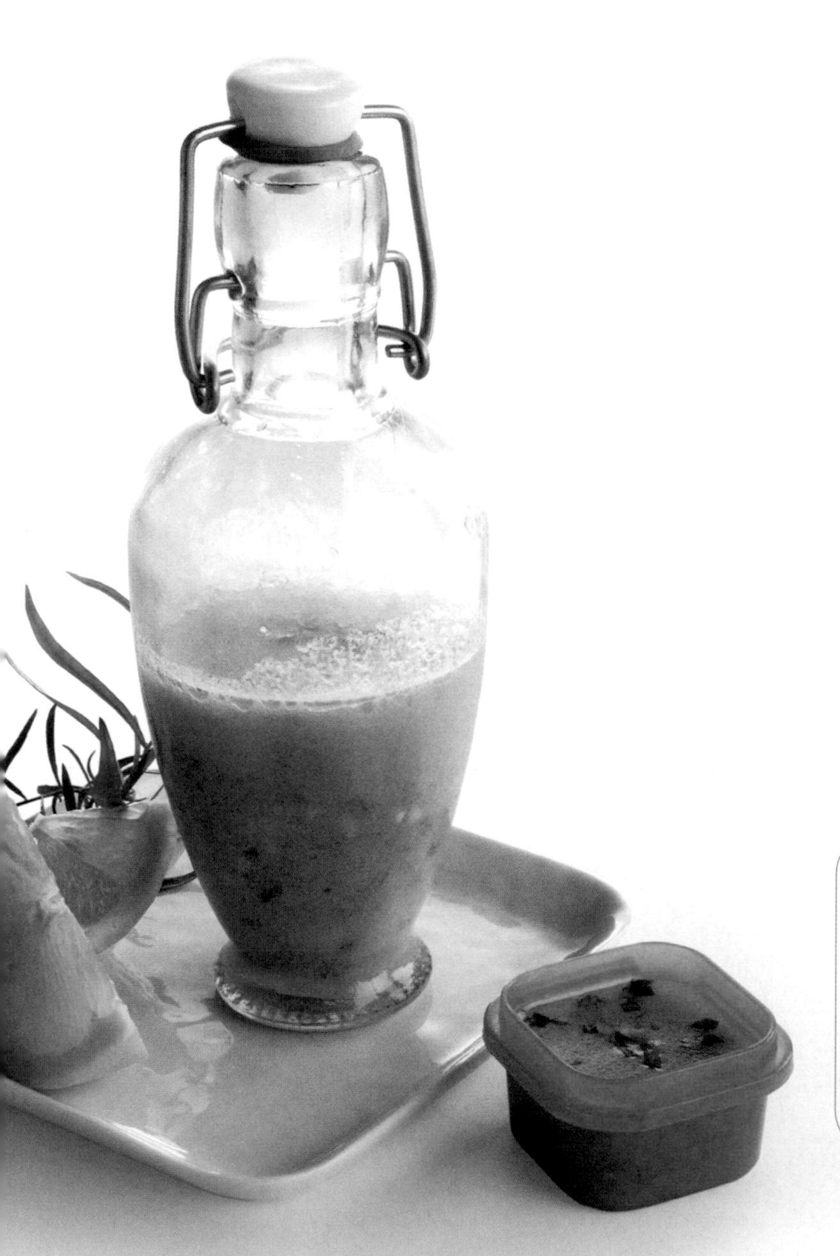

LEMON TARRAGON VINAIGRETTE

(Makes 6 servings, about 2 Tbsp. each)

Container Equivalents (per serving):
One Orange Container

¼ cup	fresh lemon juice
¼ cup	finely chopped shallot
6	fresh tarragon sprigs, leaves removed and chopped, stem discarded
4 tsp.	Dijon mustard
¼ tsp.	sea salt or Himalayan salt (Mineralize)
¼ tsp.	ground black pepper
6 Tbsp.	extra-virgin olive oil

1. Combine lemon juice, shallot, tarragon, mustard, salt, and pepper in a medium bowl; whisk to blend.
2. Slowly add oil while whisking; mix well.

TIP/SERVING SUGGESTION:
Store leftover dressing in a covered container in the refrigerator. If dressing thickens when cold, hold at room temperature for 30 minutes and stir before serving.

This dressing is wonderful on salads, but also great drizzled over sautéed veggies, steamed fish, or grilled chicken and beef.

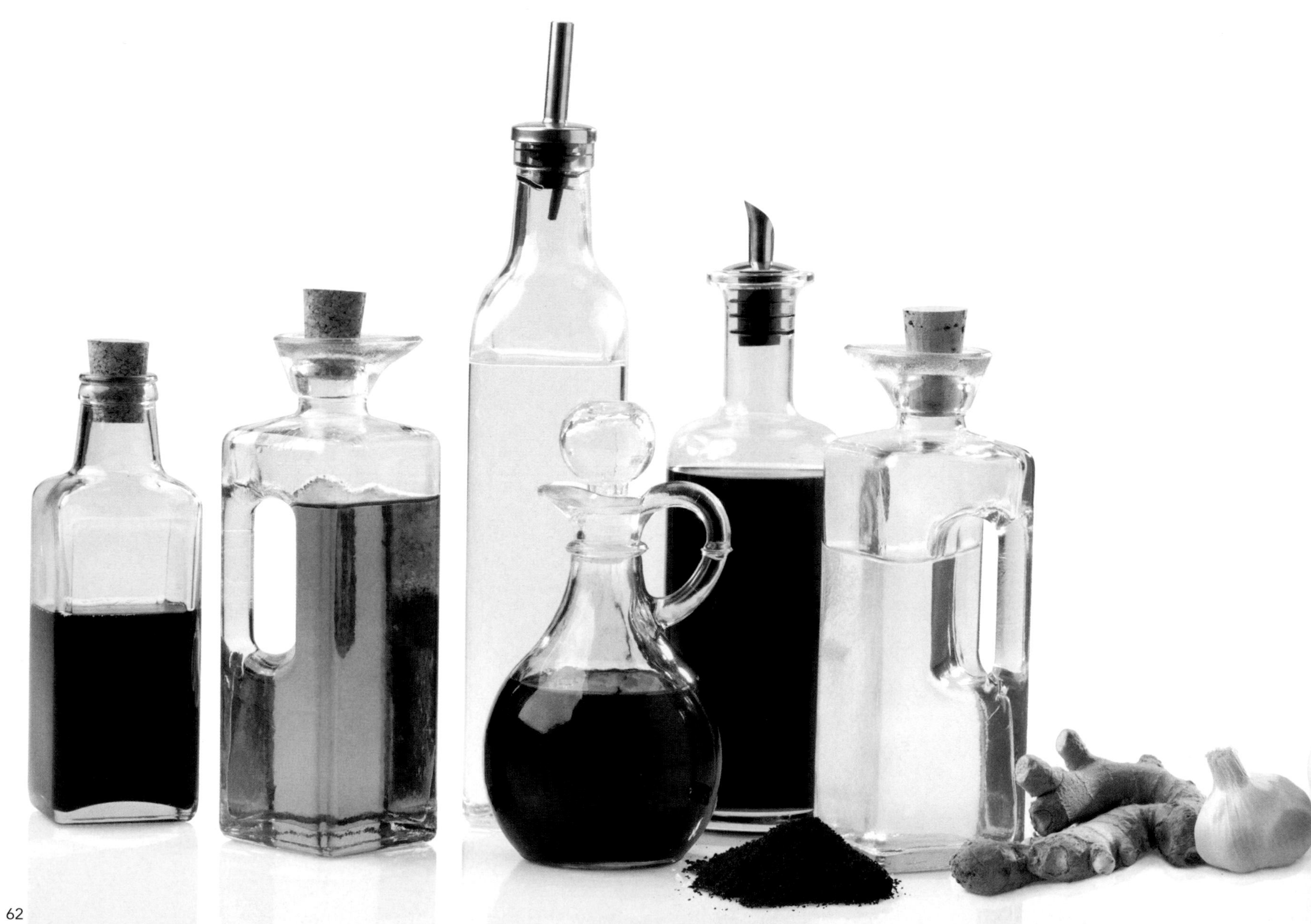

DIJON VINAIGRETTE

(Makes 8 servings, about 2 Tbsp. each)

Container Equivalents (per serving):
■ One Orange Container

3 Tbsp.	red wine vinegar
3 Tbsp.	fresh lemon juice
3 Tbsp.	Dijon mustard
2 cloves	garlic, chopped
¼ tsp.	sea salt or Himalayan salt (Mineralize)
¼ tsp.	ground black pepper
6 Tbsp.	extra-virgin olive oil

1. Combine vinegar, lemon juice, mustard, garlic, salt, and pepper in a medium bowl; whisk to blend.
2. Slowly add oil while whisking; mix well.

TIP/SERVING SUGGESTION:
Store leftover dressing in a covered container in the refrigerator. If dressing thickens when cold, hold at room temperature for 30 minutes and stir before serving.

This dressing is wonderful on salads, but also great drizzled over sautéed veggies, steamed fish, or grilled chicken, beef, and pork.

ASIAN CITRUS VINAIGRETTE

(Makes 6 servings, about 2 Tbsp. each)

Container Equivalents (per serving):
■ One Orange Container

¼ cup	100% orange juice
¼ cup	rice vinegar
2 Tbsp.	reduced-sodium soy sauce
2 tsp.	raw honey
½-inch	fresh ginger, peeled, finely grated
¼ cup	sesame oil

1. Combine orange juice, vinegar, soy sauce, honey, and ginger in a medium bowl; whisk to blend.
2. Slowly add oil while whisking; mix well.

TIP/SERVING SUGGESTION:
Store leftover dressing in a covered container in the refrigerator. If dressing thickens when cold, hold at room temperature for 30 minutes and stir before serving.

This dressing is wonderful on Asian salads or in a stir-fry, but it's also great drizzled over grilled chicken, beef, and pork.

SWEET TREATS

While these recipes are still sugary, moderation still matters. At least you know exactly what you're eating, and that these treats are Portion Fix–approved.

[NOTE: One serving of each of these treats replaces a Yellow Container portion.]

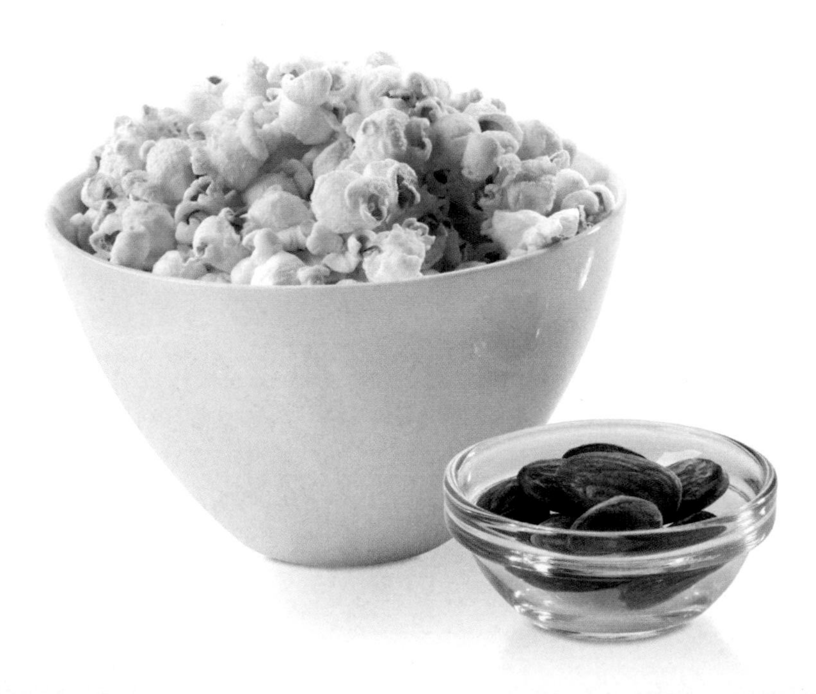

POPCORN MIX WITH RAISINS, ALMONDS, AND DRIED FRUIT

(Makes 4 servings, 1 cup each)

Container Equivalents (per serving):
One Yellow Container

3½ cups	air-popped popcorn
¼ cup	raisins
2 Tbsp.	whole raw almonds
2 Tbsp.	chopped dried fruit
½ tsp.	sea salt or Himalayan salt (Mineralize) (optional)

1. Combine popcorn, raisins, almonds, dried fruit, and salt (if desired) in a medium bowl; mix well.

TIP: Air-popped popcorn can be made using an air-popped popcorn maker (an inexpensive appliance you'll find online or at any big box retailer), or it can be made in the microwave. Place 3 Tbsp. popcorn kernels in a large brown paper bag. Seal bag tightly. Microwave on "high" for 1½ to 2 minutes or until there are 2 seconds between pops.

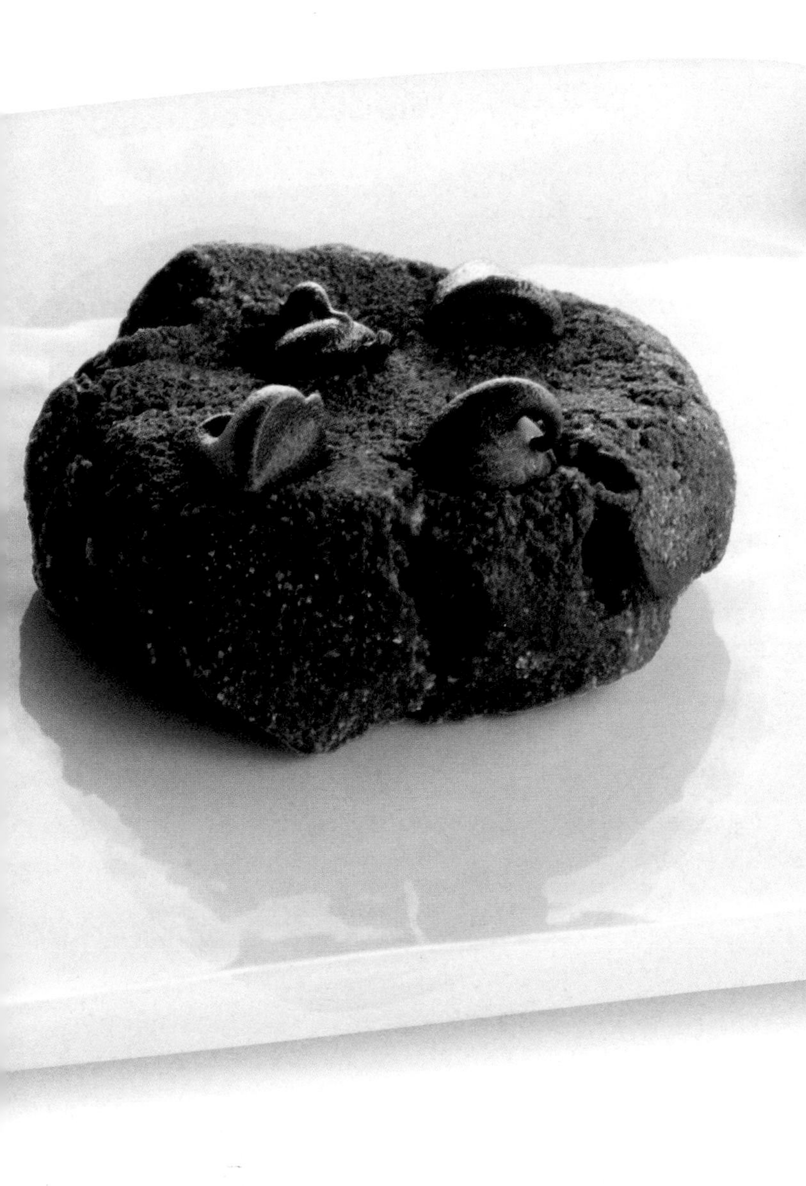

DOUBLE CHOCOLATE COOKIES

(Makes 15 servings, 1 cookie each)

Container Equivalents (per serving):
One Yellow Container

	Nonstick cooking spray
¼ cup	extra-virgin coconut oil, melted
½ cup	unsweetened applesauce
⅓ cup	pure maple syrup
¼ cup	canned lite coconut milk
⅓ cup	coconut flour
¼ cup	whole wheat flour
½ cup	all-natural cocoa powder
¼ cup	semisweet chocolate morsels (or slivered raw almonds, chopped pecans, dried cherries, or raisins)

1. Preheat oven to 350° F.
2. Lightly coat baking sheet with spray. Set aside.
3. Combine coconut oil, applesauce, maple syrup, and coconut milk in a medium bowl; mix well. Set aside.
4. Combine coconut flour, whole wheat flour, and cocoa powder in a small bowl; mix well.
5. Add flour mixture to applesauce mixture; mix until well blended.
6. Add morsels; mix until blended.
7. Drop by heaping Tbsp. onto prepared baking sheet.
8. Bake for 12 minutes or until firm.

TIP: For a gluten-free version, substitute ⅓ cup brown rice flour for whole wheat flour.

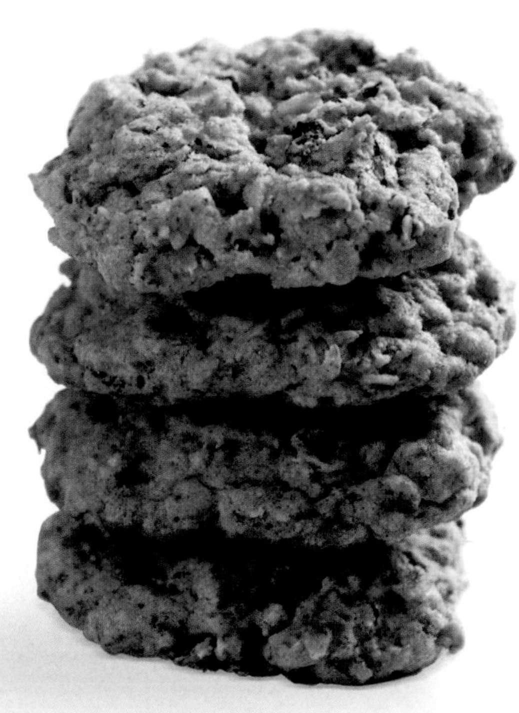

OATMEAL COOKIES WITH CHOCOLATE MORSELS AND TOASTED PECANS

(Makes 8 servings, 2 cookies each)

Container Equivalents (per serving):
One Yellow Container

	Nonstick cooking spray
1 cup	old-fashioned rolled oats
1 tsp.	ground cinnamon
¼ tsp	sea salt or Himalayan salt (Mineralize)
1 cup	unsweetened applesauce
¼ cup	semisweet chocolate morsels
¼ cup	chopped raw pecans, toasted

1. Preheat oven to 350° F.
2. Lightly coat baking sheet with spray. Set aside.
3. Combine oats, cinnamon, and salt in a medium bowl; mix well.
4. Add applesauce, morsels, and pecans; mix well.
5. Drop by heaping Tbsp. onto prepared baking sheet to form 16 cookies; flatten with a spatula.
6. Bake for 14 to 16 minutes or until firm.

HIGH-PROTEIN CHOCOLATE PEANUT BUTTER SNACK BARS

(Makes 24 servings, 1 bar each)

Container Equivalents (per serving):
One Yellow Container

4 scoops	Chocolate Shakeology
2 cups	quick-cooking old-fashioned rolled oats
⅓ cup	chopped raw peanuts
½ cup	golden raisins
1 cup	unsweetened almond milk
½ cup	all-natural creamy peanut butter

1. Combine Shakeology, oats, peanuts, and raisins in a large mixing bowl; mix well.
2. Add almond milk and peanut butter; mix well.
3. Press mixture into 8 x 8-inch baking pan; cover and refrigerate for at least 3 hours.
4. Cut into 24 bars.

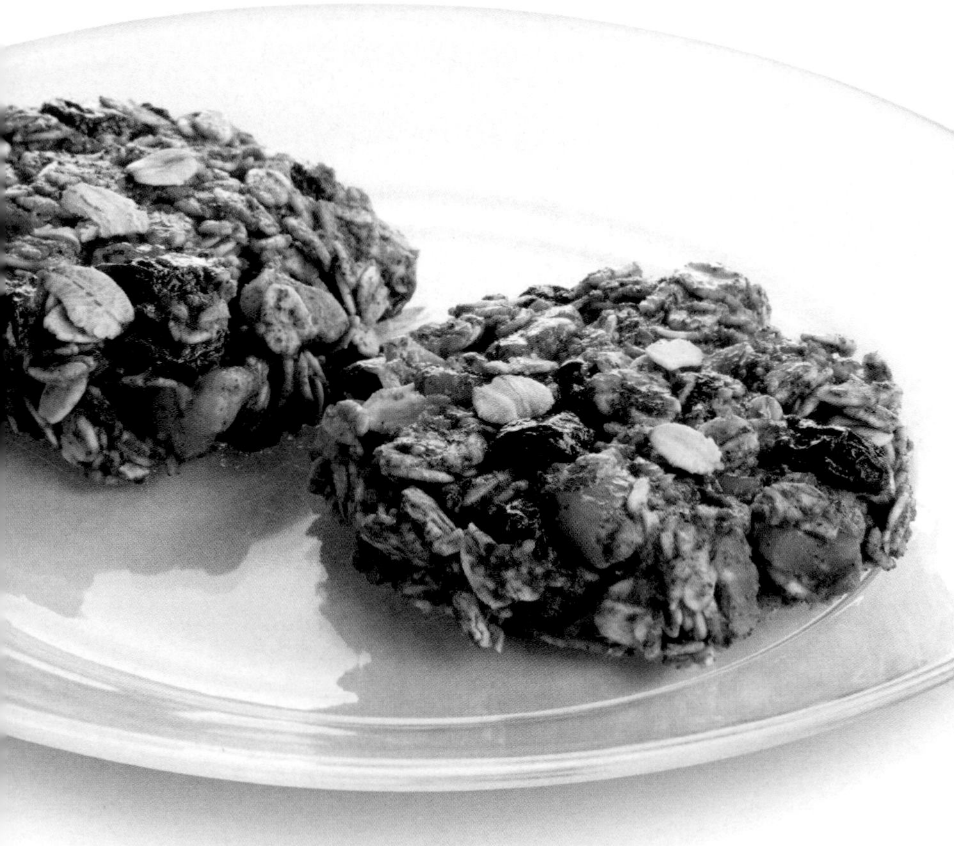

BANANA OATMEAL COOKIES

(Makes 8 servings, 2 cookies each)

Container Equivalents (per serving):
One Yellow Container

	Nonstick cooking spray
1 cup	old-fashioned rolled oats
2 tsp.	ground cinnamon
¼ tsp.	sea salt or Himalayan salt (Mineralize)
2	ripe medium bananas, mashed
¼ cup	golden raisins
¼ cup	chopped raw walnuts

1. Preheat oven to 350° F.
2. Lightly coat baking sheet with spray. Set aside.
3. Combine oats, cinnamon, and salt in a medium bowl; mix well.
4. Add bananas, raisins, and walnuts; mix well.
5. Drop by heaping Tbsp. onto prepared baking sheet to form 16 cookies; flatten with a spatula.
6. Bake for 14 to 15 minutes or until firm.

SHAKEOLOGY

This shake is formulated unlike any other shake you have ever tried. Made from superfoods harvested from around the globe—Shakeology provides ALL the supernutrients you need—phytonutrients, antioxidants, enzymes, pre- and probiotics, fiber, adaptogens, vitamins, and minerals.

This is quite likely the healthiest thing you will consume. Truly. You'll feel more energized, you'll become regular, and it is clinically proven to aid weight loss! Drink it daily. Your body, your health will love this shake.*

CHOCOLATE CHAI

(Makes 1 serving)

Container Equivalents (per serving):
■ One Red Container

8 fl oz	brewed black tea, cooled
1 scoop	Chocolate Shakeology
¼ tsp.	pumpkin pie spice
8 fl oz	ice

Place tea, Shakeology, pumpkin pie spice, and ice in blender; cover. Blend until smooth.

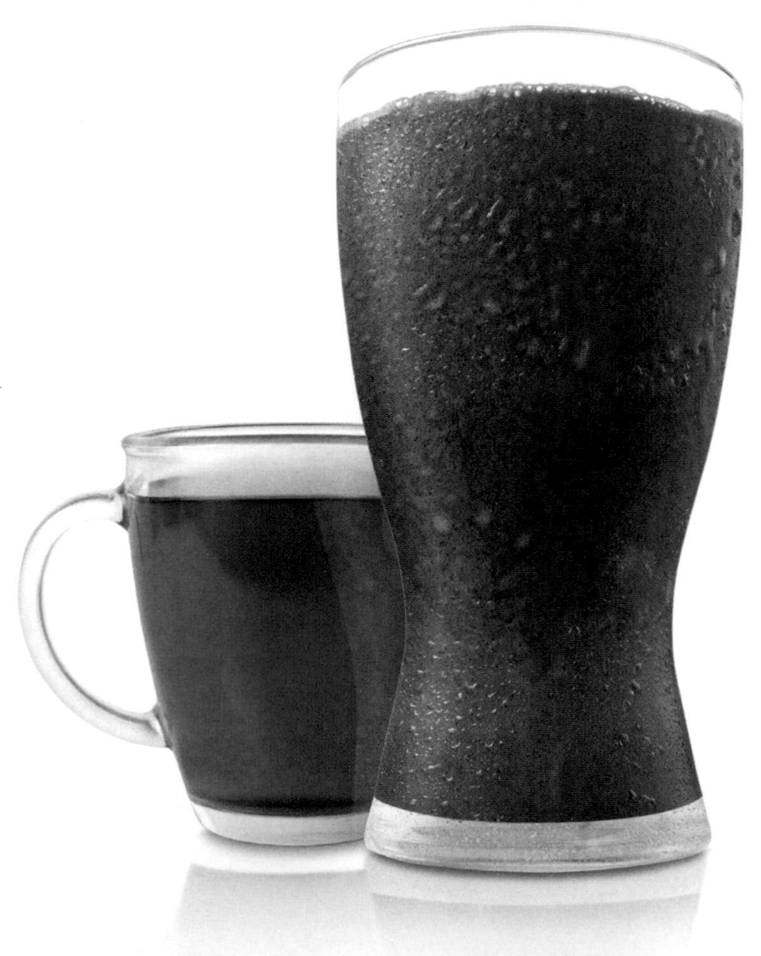

*Results vary. Results based on a twelve-week independent clinical trial sponsored by Beachbody, where fifty people consumed Shakeology as their breakfast and lunch with no other changes to their diet or exercise regimen. These statements have not been evaluated by the Food and Drug Administration. This product is not intended to diagnose, treat, cure, or prevent any disease.

VANILLA MOCHA

(Makes 1 serving)

Container Equivalents (per serving):
■ One Red Container

8 fl oz	brewed unsweetened coffee, cooled
1 scoop	Chocolate Shakeology
½ tsp.	pure vanilla extract
8 fl oz	ice

Place coffee, Shakeology, extract, and ice in blender; cover. Blend until smooth.

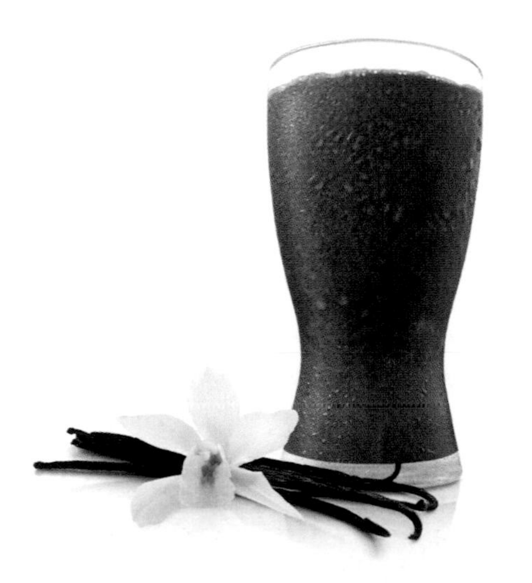

VANILLA CHAI

(Makes 1 serving)

Container Equivalents (per serving):
■ One Red Container

4 fl oz	brewed unsweetened chai tea, cooled
4 fl oz	water
1 scoop	Vanilla Shakeology
1 dash	ground allspice
8 fl oz	ice

Place tea, water, Shakeology, allspice, and ice in blender; cover. Blend until smooth.

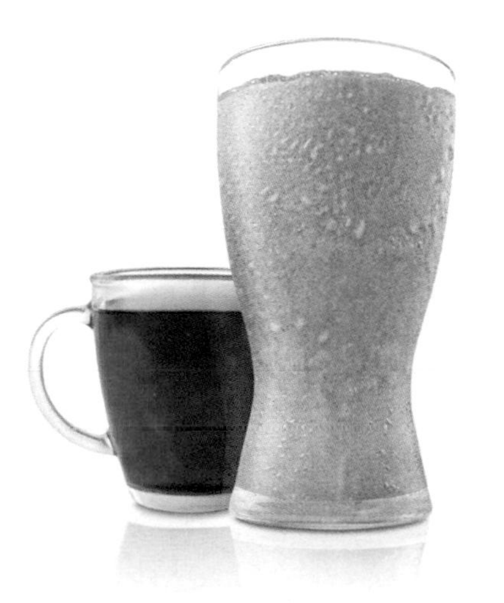

STRAWBERRY MOJITO

(Makes 1 serving)

Container Equivalents (per serving):
■ One Red Container

8 fl oz	water
1 scoop	Strawberry or Tropical Strawberry Vegan Shakeology
3 tsp.	fresh lime juice
6 tsp.	chopped fresh mint leaves
8 fl oz	ice

Place water, Shakeology, lime juice, mint leaves, and ice in blender; cover. Blend until smooth.

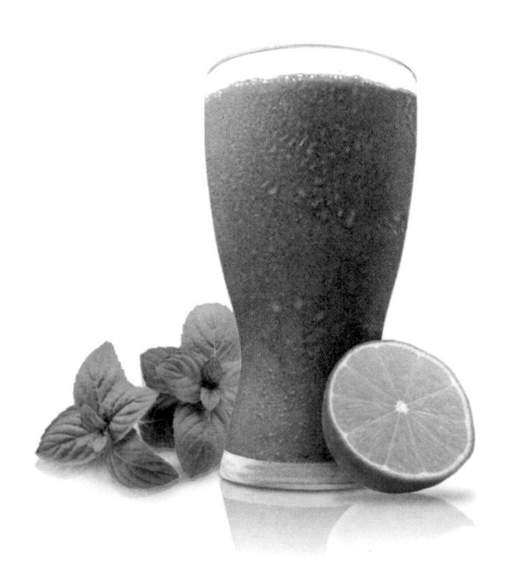

BASIL DELIGHT

(Makes 1 serving)

Container Equivalents (per serving):
■ One Red Container

8 fl oz	water
1 scoop	Greenberry Shakeology
3 tsp.	fresh lime juice
6 tsp.	chopped fresh basil leaves
8 fl oz	ice

Place water, Shakeology, lime juice, basil, and ice in blender; cover. Blend until smooth.

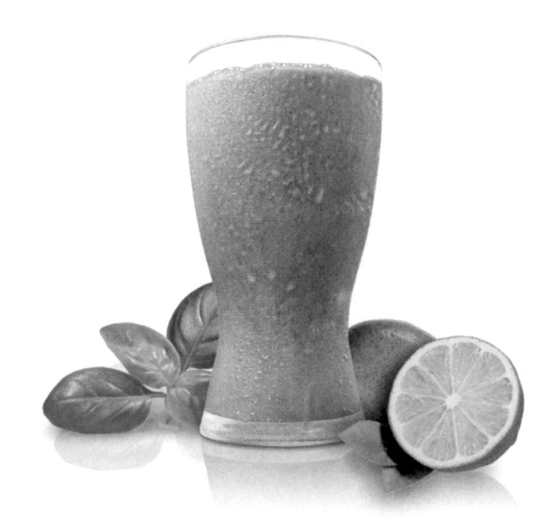

PB & B

(Makes 1 serving)

Container Equivalents (per serving):
One Red Container and
Three Teaspoons

8 fl oz	water
1 scoop	Chocolate Shakeology
3 tsp.	all-natural peanut butter, almond butter, or any nut butter
¼	medium banana
8 fl oz	ice

Place water, Shakeology, peanut butter, banana, and ice in blender; cover. Blend until smooth.

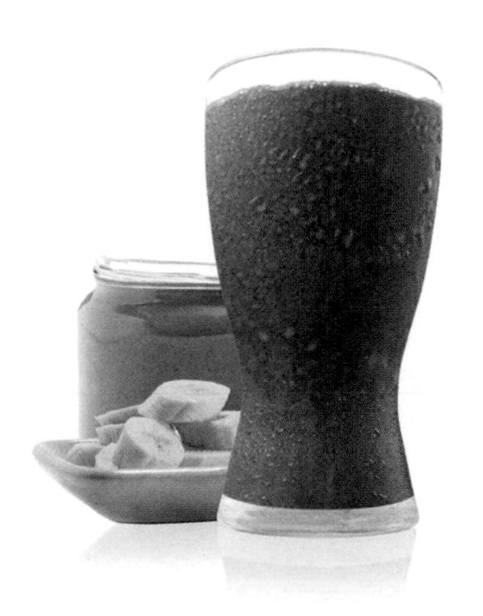

PB & J

(Makes 1 serving)

Container Equivalents (per serving):
One Red Container,
One Purple Container, and
Two Teaspoons

8 fl oz	water
1 scoop	Chocolate Shakeology
1 cup	red grapes
2 tsp.	all-natural peanut butter, almond butter, or any nut butter
8 fl oz	ice

Place water, Shakeology, grapes, peanut butter, and ice in blender; cover. Blend until smooth.

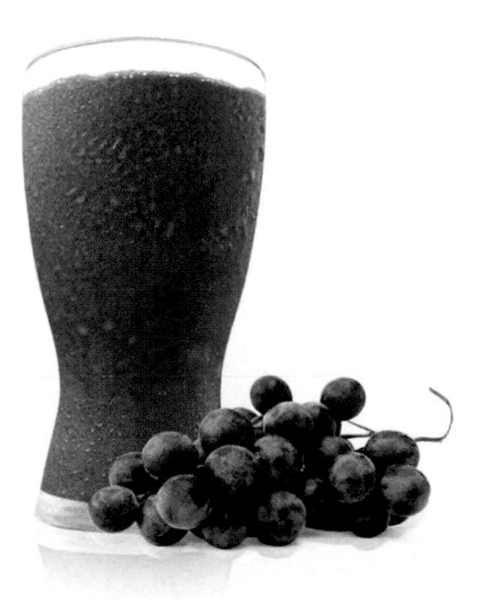

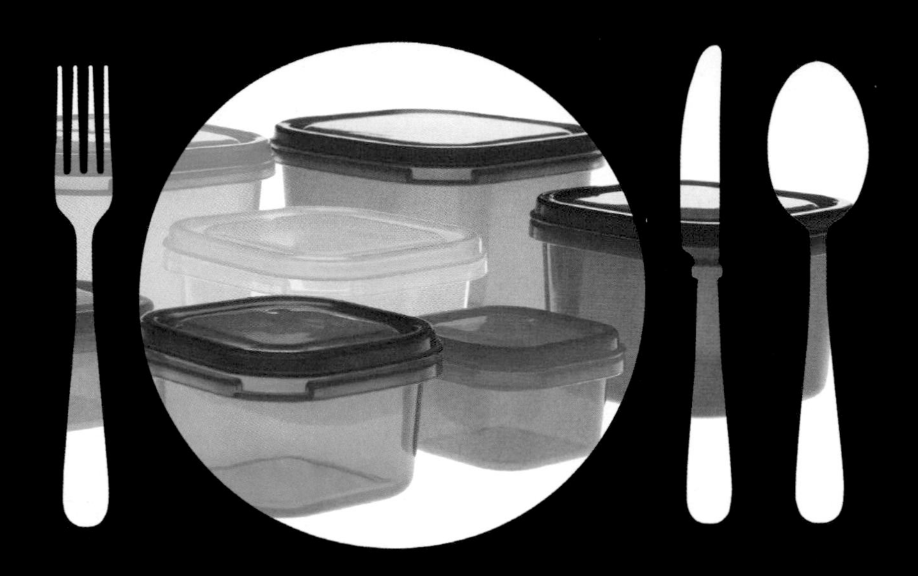

SAMPLE PORTION PLAN

The Portion Fix gives you plenty of freedom, but sometimes it's helpful to see an actual real-life example of how things can be put together. So here are three days of how someone might eat on the plan. Just pick out the meals that interest you, then consult page 11 to see how many containers of each you need for your Portion Plan. These meal times are just suggestions. Obviously, you'll need to work with your schedule to find the times that work best for you.

Remember, the colored dots indicate which container group these foods come from, but not the amount you should eat. The [teaspoon icon] indicates the teaspoon group. No dot at all indicates a FREE FOOD.

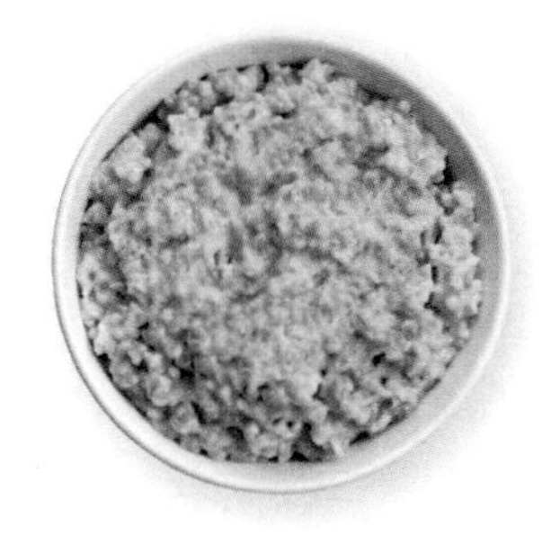

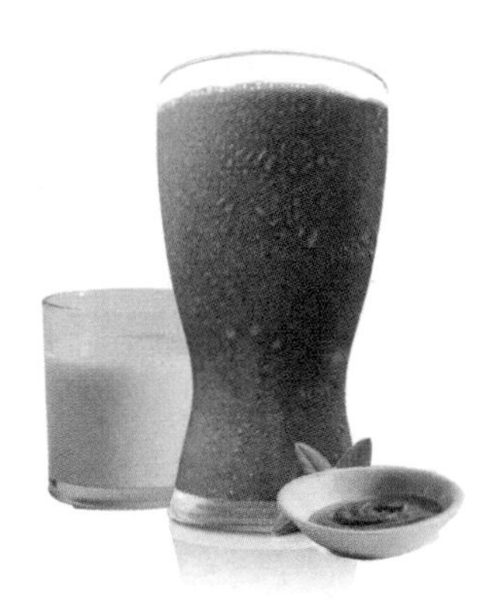

7:00 AM | BREAKFAST: CHOOSE ONE

- Hard-boiled eggs
- Cooked oatmeal, steel-cut with ground cinnamon
- Sliced apples

—— OR ——

- 1% Greek yogurt sprinkled with cinnamon
- Cereal, whole-grain
- Blueberries

—— OR ——

- Turkey bacon
- Whole-grain bread
- Strawberries

10:00 AM | SNACK 1 – SHAKEOLOGY: CHOOSE ONE

- Water
- Shakeology
- Natural peanut or almond butter

—— OR ——

- Water
- Shakeology
- Avocado
- Coconut extract

—— OR ——

- Water
- Shakeology
- Sunflower seed butter
- Ground cinnamon

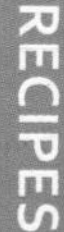

12:30 PM I **LUNCH:** CHOOSE ONE

- Mixed salad (lettuce, cucumbers, tomatoes, bell peppers)
- Grilled chicken breast cooked in olive oil and sprinkled with a Seasoning Mix
- Cooked quinoa

—— OR ——

- Grilled salmon cooked in olive oil and sprinkled with a Seasoning Mix
- Roasted asparagus topped with sesame seeds
- Sliced carrots
- Cooked lentils sprinkled with dried oregano

—— OR ——

- Grilled tempeh cooked in olive oil and sprinkled with a Seasoning Mix
- Steamed snow peas
- Steamed broccoli sprinkled with a Seasoning Mix
- Cooked brown rice topped with sunflower seeds and sprinkled with chopped fresh cilantro

3:30 PM I **SNACK 2:** CHOOSE ONE

- Raw whole almonds

—— OR ——

- Hummus spread on a lettuce leaf

—— OR ——

- Avocado drizzled with balsamic vinegar

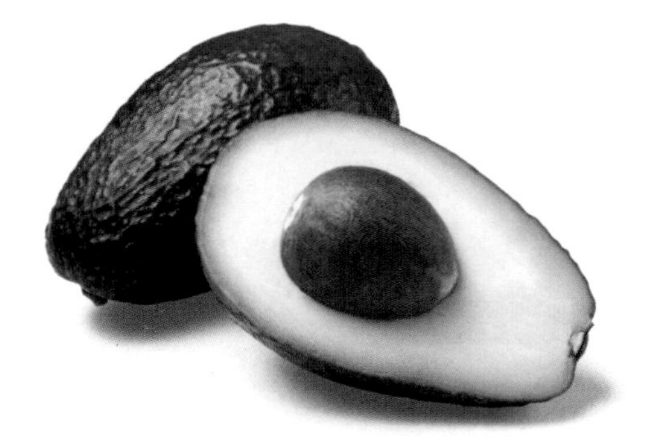

6:00 PM | DINNER: CHOOSE ONE

- Grilled flank steak using a Seasoning Mix as a rub
- Cooked carrots with smoked paprika

—— OR ——

- Grilled chicken breast sprinkled with a Seasoning Mix
- Steamed kale sprinkled with a Seasoning Mix

—— OR ——

- Grilled veggie burger patty sprinkled with a Seasoning Mix
- Steamed summer squash (zucchini) sprinkled with a Seasoning Mix

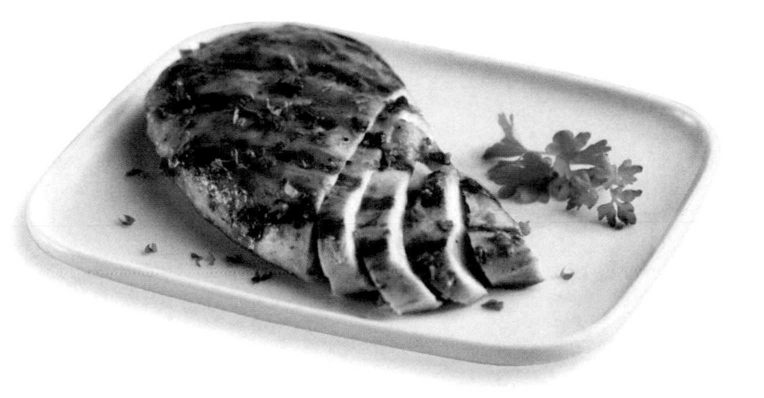

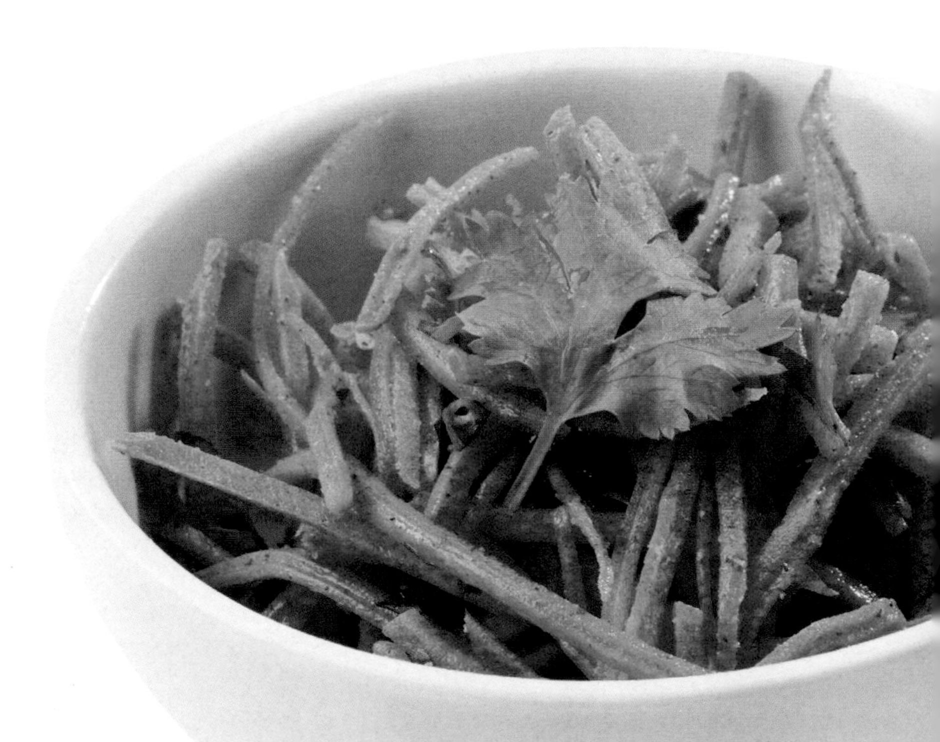

DISCOVER OTHER HIT PRODUCTS FROM BEACHBODY®!

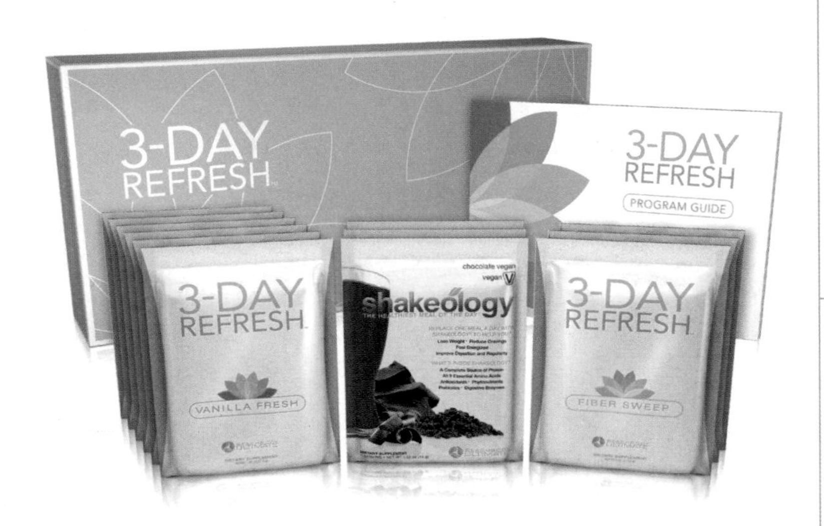

3-DAY REFRESH®

Feel leaner and cleaner—WITHOUT starving! If you're looking for a way to lose a few pounds quickly, improve digestion, and feel more energized, then the **3-Day Refresh** is for you.*

Retail Price $69.95
Club Price $62.96
Coach Price $52.46

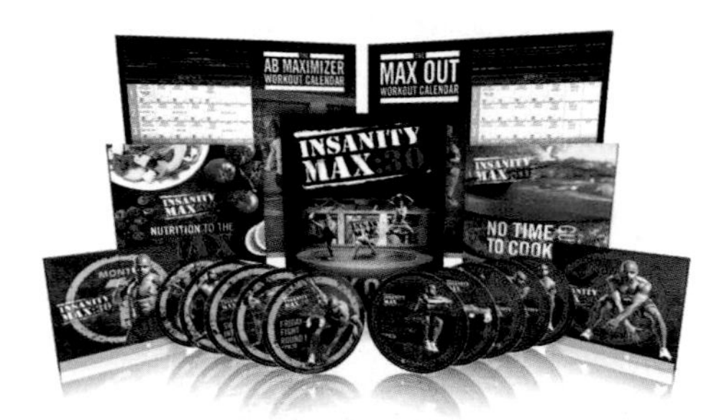

INSANITY MAX:30™

MAX OUT for MAX results! With **INSANITY MAX:30**, the only thing standing between you and the body you want . . . is YOU. Just push to your personal MAX and get insane results in 30 minutes a day.

Retail Price $119.85
Club Price $107.87
Coach Price $89.89

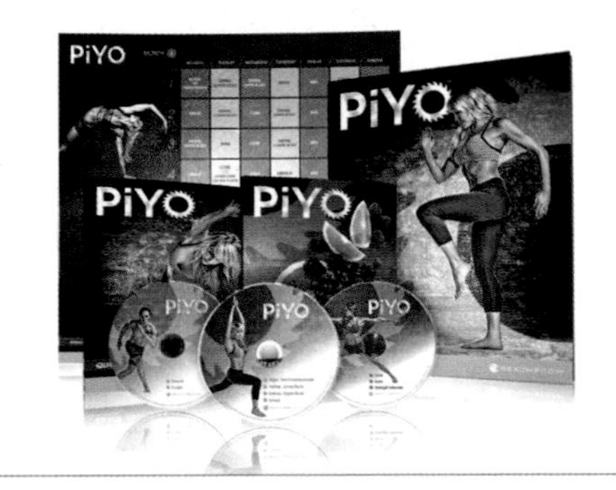

PiYo®

Define every inch of your body without bulking up or straining your joints. **PiYo** is a low-impact workout that gives you strength training, flexibility, and cardio—all at once!

Retail Price $59.85
Club Price $53.87
Coach Price $44.89

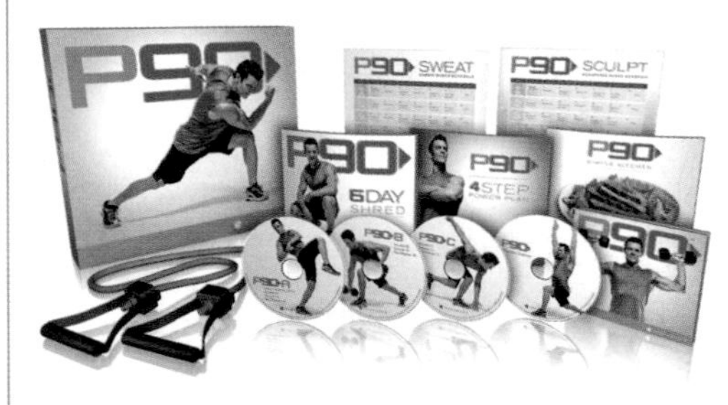

P90®

Now you don't have to go to the extreme to get dramatic, visible results! **P90** is the program YOU can do. With workouts that are simple, doable, and less extreme, this is fitness for EVERY BODY.

Retail Price $79.90
Club Price $71.91
Coach Price $59.93

AVAILABLE THROUGH YOUR TEAM BEACHBODY COACH OR AT BEACHBODY.COM.

*These statements have not been evaluated by the Food and Drug Administration. These products are not intended to diagnose, treat, cure, or prevent any disease.

All prices and products shown are subject to change. Please visit Beachbody.com for the most current information.

GET A FREE COACH TO HELP YOU SUCCEED!

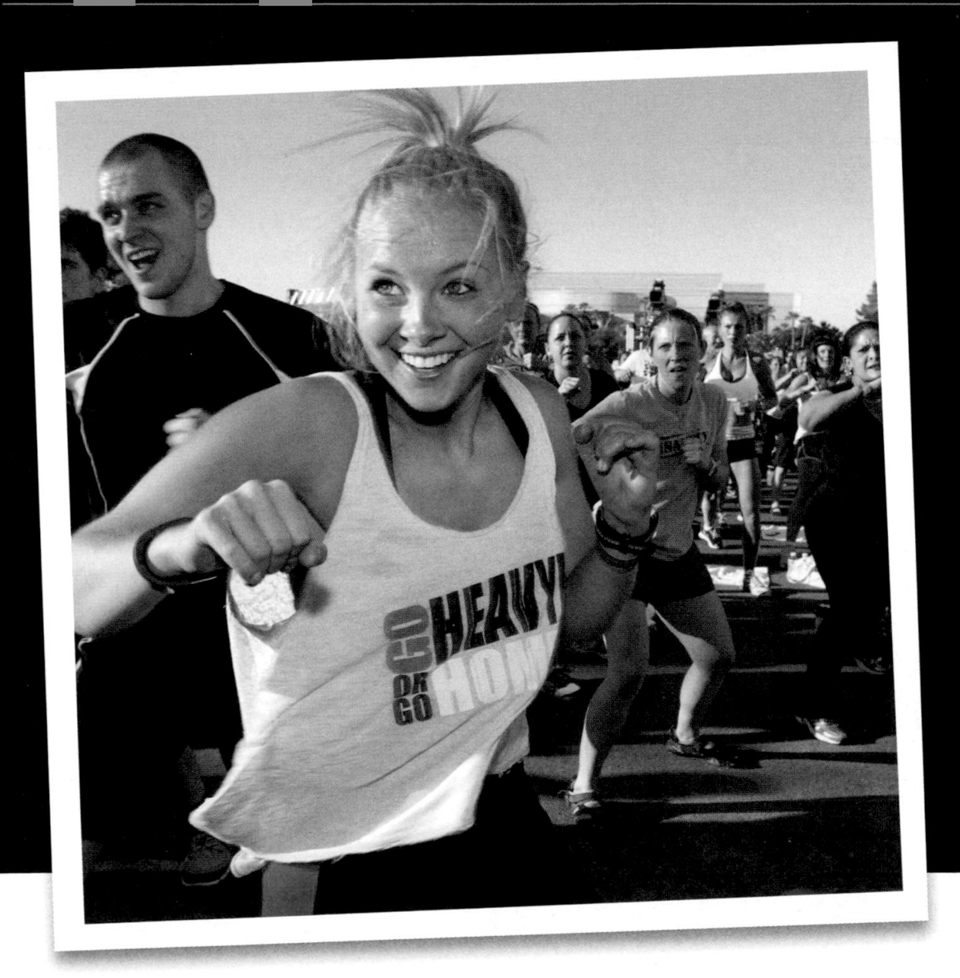

What's a Team Beachbody Coach?

A COACH IS A CUSTOMER, JUST LIKE YOU, who has seen great results from using Beachbody products and wants to help you reach your goals.

How can a Coach help?

YOUR COACH WILL HELP KEEP YOU MOTIVATED, and stay in touch, online or over the phone. They'll also set you up on TeamBeachbody.com for the best nutrition and exercise tips.

And here's the best part:

IT'S FREE. IT COSTS YOU ABSOLUTELY NOTHING. Millions of people have partnered with their Coaches to achieve their dream bodies.

SO WHAT ARE YOU WAITING FOR?
You can do this!

Get your Coach today at
GETMYFREECOACH.COM

One scoop of Shakeology® is the perfect portion for a much healthier you.

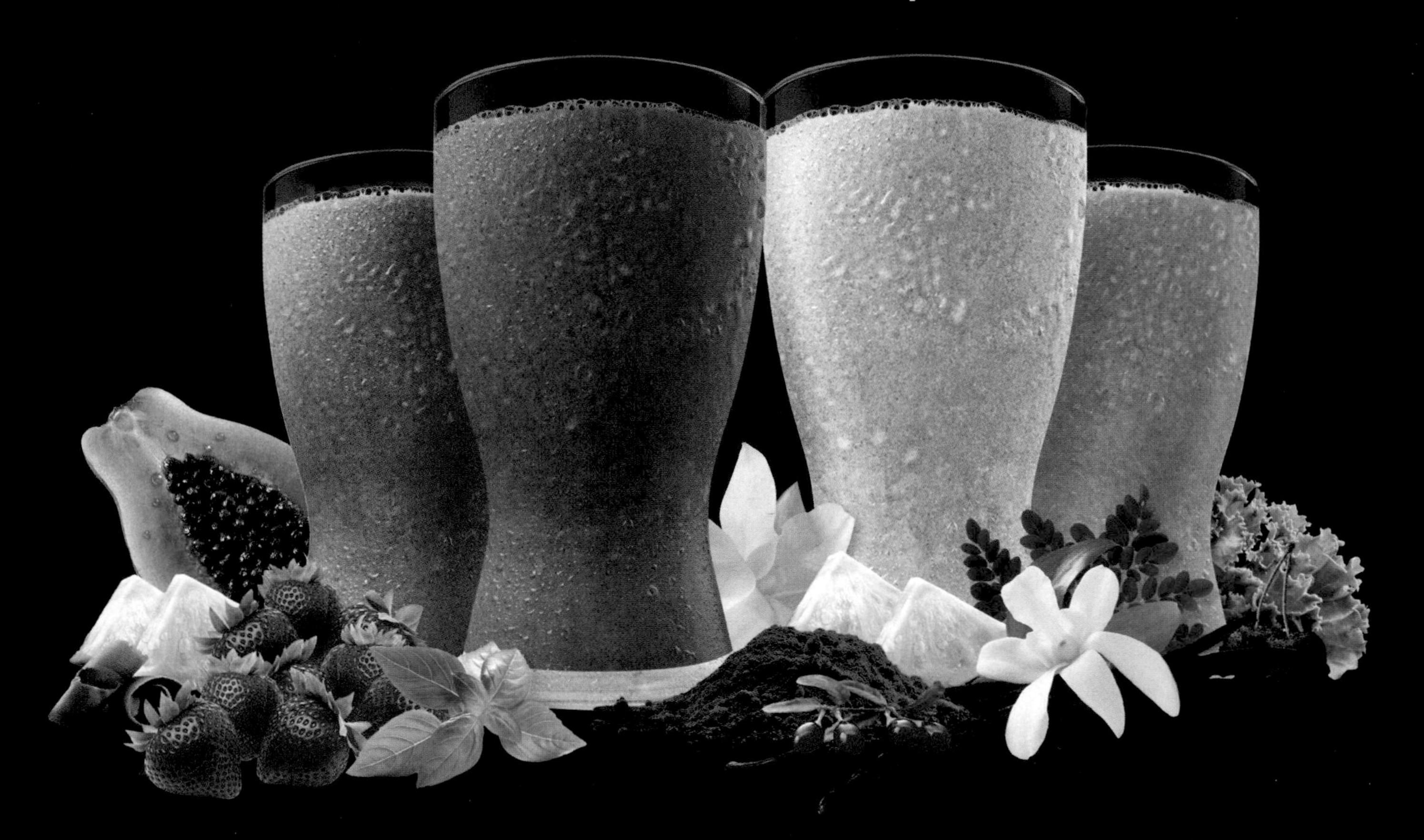

NOW AVAILABLE IN 6 DELICIOUS FLAVORS:

Vanilla • Chocolate • Strawberry • Greenberry • Tropical Strawberry Vegan • Chocolate Vegan

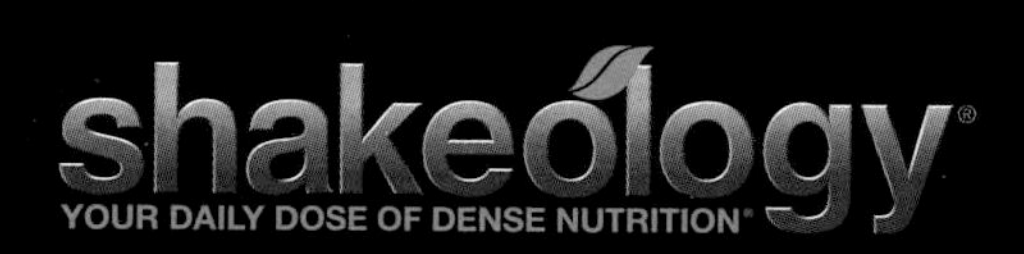

Shakeology helps curb cravings.†

The amazing thing about Shakeology is that my food cravings are gone. I don't crave fast food, chips, candy bars, or anything like that anymore.

—David G., Oklahoma

Shakeology helps you lose weight.†

I knew I needed to lose weight but was struggling to quit drinking diet soda. I replaced the diet soda with Shakeology as my treat for the day. I haven't had a diet soda since the day I started Shakeology! And I've lost 18 pounds so far.

—Susan T., Washington

The Portion Fix was specifically designed to include Shakeology as an easy and super-satisfying way to help you get maximum weight-loss results.*

This shake is formulated unlike any other shake you have ever tried. Made from superfoods harvested from around the globe—Shakeology provides the supernutrients your body craves—phytonutrients, antioxidants, enzymes, pre- and probiotics, fiber, adaptogens, vitamins, and minerals. This is quite likely the healthiest thing you will ever consume. Truly. You'll feel more energized, you'll become more regular, and it is clinically proven to help aid weight loss!* Drink it daily. Your body, your health will love this shake.†

According to a survey of nearly 3,000 daily Shakeology drinkers:**

- **93%** feel healthier since drinking it.
- **81%** feel it has helped them reduce their cravings for junk food.
- **86%** experience an increase in their energy levels.
- **97%** feel Shakeology is a smart investment in their health.

It's our Bottom-of-the-Bag Guarantee.

We're so sure Shakeology will improve your health, we've created an amazing guarantee. Try Shakeology for 30 days and if you don't feel healthier, return it and we'll refund your money (less s&h). Even if the bag is totally empty.

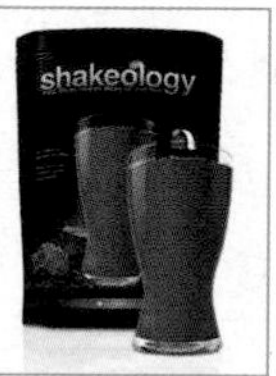

To learn more, contact your Team Beachbody® Coach or visit ShakeologyPortionFix.com today.

FOLLOW SHAKEOLOGY ON:

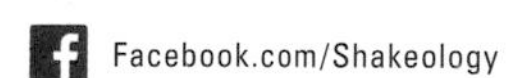
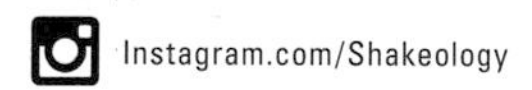
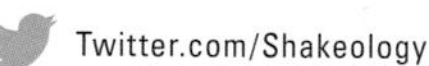
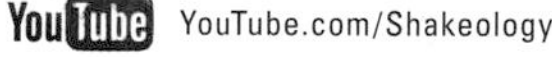
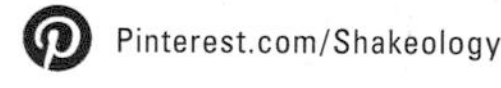

Facebook.com/Shakeology Instagram.com/Shakeology Twitter.com/Shakeology YouTube.com/Shakeology Pinterest.com/Shakeology

*Results vary. Results based on a twelve-week independent clinical trial sponsored by Beachbody, where fifty people consumed Shakeology as their breakfast and lunch with no other changes to their diet or exercise regimen.

†These statements have not been evaluated by the Food and Drug Administration. This product is not intended to diagnose, treat, cure, or prevent any disease.

**Based on a survey of 2,769 Shakeology users who drank Shakeology 5 or more times per week and exercised 3 times per week.

TEAM BEACHBODY CLUB

LET'S LOSE WEIGHT TOGETHER.

Your purchase of **Portion Fix** is the first step to learning simple portion control—and finally losing the weight! However, to get the best results from this nutrition plan, you also need great support, real accountability, and the daily commitment to working out and eating healthy. That's where the Team Beachbody VIP Club Membership comes in. It's an essential tool for staying on track and achieving your goals!

VIP access to TeamBeachbody.com gives you everything you need to increase your success with Portion Fix:

1. Personalized online meal plans based on your individual goals
2. Diet and workout advice from fitness and nutrition experts
3. Nutrition tools, including a Healthy Weight Calculator and Body Fat Calculator
4. Message Boards where you can get answers to all your food and fitness questions 24/7
5. A FREE Coach for questions, concerns, or just a bit of encouragement along the way
6. **10% discount on Shakeology, fitness programs, gear, and supplements with a paid Team Beachbody Club membership**

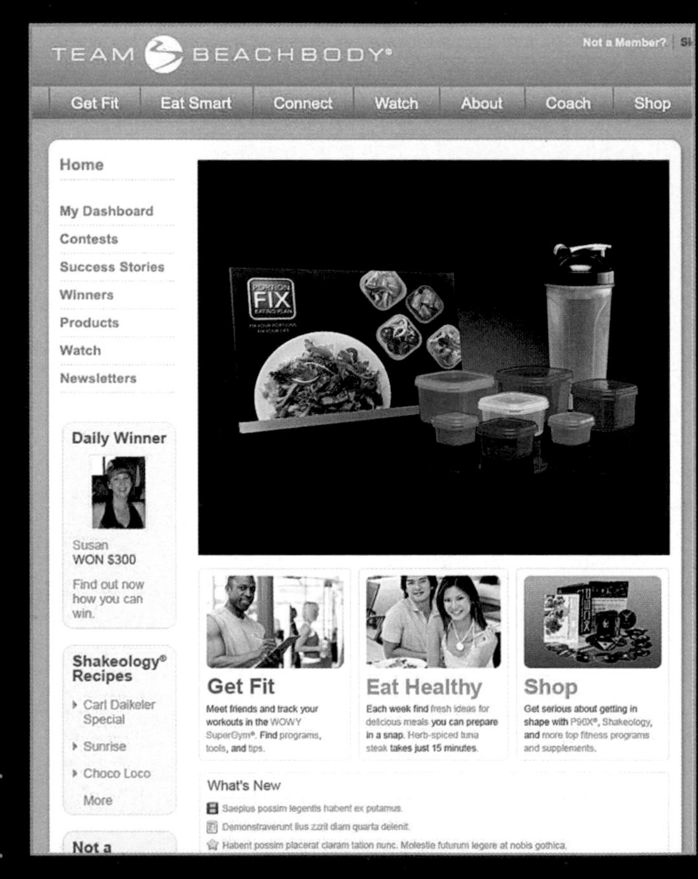

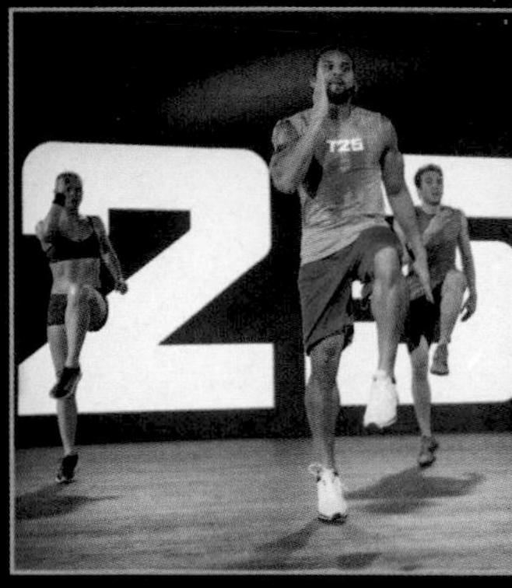

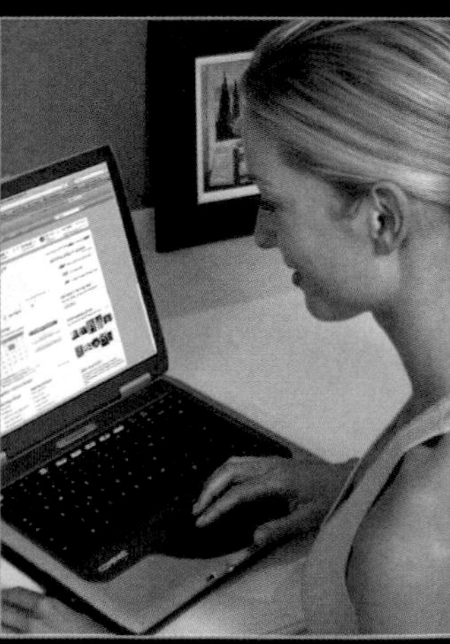

To gain VIP access, sign up for your RISK-FREE 30-DAY TRIAL at **TEAMBEACHBODY.COM/SIGNUP**

▶ **Act now and get a FREE GIFT!**